Leo Angart

magic eyes
vision training for children

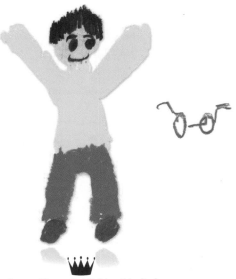

Crown House Publishing Limited
www.crownhouse.co.uk
www.crownhousepublishing.com

First published by

Crown House Publishing Ltd
Crown Buildings, Bancyfelin, Carmarthen,
Wales, SA33 5ND, UK
www.crownhouse.co.uk

and

Crown House Publishing Company LLC
6 Trowbridge Drive, Suite 5, Bethel, CT 06801, USA
www.crownhousepublishing.com

First published 2015.

British Library Cataloguing-in-Publication Data
A catalogue entry for this book is available
from the British Library.

Print ISBN 978-184590959-8
Mobi ISBN 978-184590964-2
ePub ISBN 978-184590965-9
ePDF ISBN 978-184590966-6
LCCN 2015933289

Printed and bound in the UK by
Bell & Bain Ltd, Thornliebank, Glasgow

DISCLAIMER

Magic Eyes is not meant for diagnosis and treatment for any medical condition for the eye or the visual system. The author, publisher and distributor are in no way liable for any damage whatsoever arising from the use or misuse of this material or the exercises suggested including but not limited to any personal injury. If you are in any doubt contact your doctor.

Acknowledgments

First I wish to thank the pioneers of vision training. Most of all William H. Bates, M.D., who in the early 1900s realized that vision problems are functional and can therefore be improved with exercises. Another pioneer is Arthur M. Skeffington, M.D. who in 1928 co-founded the Optometric Extension Program. Skeffington believed that vision is a function of many parts including how we perceive what's seen.

Without the achievements of the many kids in my workshops this book would not be possible. What works has emerged over 20 years of play with children in Magic Eyes workshops around the world.

Long ago I realized that many people had suffered vision problems that could, in most cases, easily have been corrected when they were children. For example, a man in his sixties told me that he could only read one word at a time. In the workshop for adults we discovered that his eyes were focusing 15 cm above the book he was trying to read. With the eye co-ordination exercise described in this book he was able to read again naturally. He told me that he wished we had met 50 years earlier. My dream is that all children will benefit from the tests and exercises in this book and grow up with "Magic Eyes."

I also want to thank the many people who helped make this book possible. Eva Maria Spitzer who researched and checked everything, thank you Eva. Gökçen Eke who created the cute cartoons that illustrate this book. Wolfgang Gillessen for his support with all my books.

Finally I also want to thank the team at Crown House Publishing for bringing this book to you.

Leo Angart

Contents

1. Introduction

Magic Eyes and the eyesight of children are topics very close to my heart. For more than 18 years I have worked extensively with children all over the world. My primary work is the restoration of children's eyesight by natural means – that is, without glasses, lenses, surgery or expensive therapy sessions.

Early on, I realized that I personally cannot restore someone else's eyesight for them. It is something every individual has to do for themselves. However, with children it is actually easier, for a number of reasons. Primarily, children are already at a developmental stage where their bodies, minds and eyesight are in the process of change. If training is done in a simple way, then its purpose is simply the restoration of the natural path of development.

The first stage is to remove, or counteract, the cause of any visual problem. However, before you can embark on this, it is important to have a good understanding of the child's condition. For instance, in order to be able to help their child, parents should be well-informed about the main causes of near-sight and the way that poor eye co-ordination can affect learning in a dysfunctional way.

In my travels I have met many wonderful kids and young people, but I have often been saddened when they present problems that could have been detected and corrected early on. For example, in one of my workshops, a young man realized why he had never been able to read for more than 30 minutes before it became too painful to carry on. He discovered that his point of convergence was an arm's length in front of him. No wonder attempting to read anything closer than that was very stressful! After this situation was redressed, he exclaimed, with joy in his voice, "Now I can read a novel for pleasure!" His problem should have been detected in kindergarten or, at the very latest, in primary school; not 20 years later in my workshop.

Most professional eye-care practitioners have a different view of vision and the way that the eyes work. Their training usually does not include the notion that you can rehabilitate the visual system as easily as other systems in the body. However, in more recent years the concept of brain plasticity has become more popular. This modality takes for granted the ability of the brain to relearn and postulates that it is always taking in new information and adapting to changing environments.

This book is written as an attempt to help parents get involved in improving their children's eyesight. I believe in the power of parents to make things happen. I have described various visual phenomena, as well as ways to detect them. And, most importantly, I have incorporated some simple exercises that parents can do with their child at home. I have also included references to scientific studies in order to broaden parents' understanding.

Introduction

It is my hope that mothers and fathers will use the information in this book to check whether their children have mastered the necessary visual skills for effective learning. If not, then they can initiate the exercises themselves and in most cases it will make a big difference to their children's eyesight. Of course, professional help may be needed as well. If this is necessary, then parents will be much more knowledgeable about their child's condition and the various treatment options available.

Vision Training is not rocket science. It is based on simple common-sense principles. Children are eager learners and will take to these exercises like ducks to water. My approach, as outlined in this book, differs from most optometric vision training which employs optics and various pieces of equipment. This generally involves regular sessions over several months. My approach goes much further and treats many more conditions, including myopia, hyperopia, astigmatism, amblyopia, eye co-ordination and strabismus.

I like to take advantage of parental love! This training is something that parents and children can do together. In this setting, in the comfort of the family home, parents can keep increasing the number of exercises and thus get results fast. The brain learns very quickly. It takes only a few seconds to register a phobia but much longer to let go of it.

The physical element of the visual system is operated by muscles, so visual training resembles any other skill training. The more you practice, the better you perform. With children, the key is to keep them motivated by making it fun and exciting.

Thankfully, kids usually get excited by their own progress and go for it full force.

This book is not an attempt to minimize or circumvent professional practices. There are limits to what parents can do on their own. The real purpose is to raise awareness about these issues and help to find solutions for affected children before they become labeled as deficient.

It is my dream that one day there will be dedicated Vision Training professionals with an eclectic approach who will take the best bits that work from all the varied disciplines available. All too often progress is limited or stalled because of commercial interests. I happen to think that helping a child to reach their full potential is priceless. What an achievement it can be to help an 8-year-old gain control of the way his eyes move, so he can read or play basketball. This will make a huge difference to the rest of this boy's life. And, in the end, that is what makes life worthwhile.

2. How to Use This Book

This book contains a lot of information. The abundance of new words and concepts may make it a challenging read. My suggestion is that you start off by dipping into the section that drew you to buy the book in the first place.

For example, if your child is becoming near-sighted, then go to the section about myopia. Take the measurement as described and discover what kind of near-sight your child has. Then you can get going with the child on the exercises I describe.

On the other hand, if you do not know exactly what the problem is, then I suggest you start at the beginning. In this way, you will not only increase your knowledge about vision, but you will also gain an insight into how it relates to a child's ability to learn. You may like to perform some of the tests and exercises described with your child as you go along. You can then eliminate many possible visual conditions by observing which tests your child can accomplish with ease.

Next, it is important to make sure that there are no visual efficiency issues, such as eye co-ordination, eye movement or focusing problems. This informs us whether the basic physical system is functioning as it should. For example, there should be no input problems (as described in Chapter 6 on visual efficiency). Fitting glasses does not do anything for these problems. The typical vision test performed in schools only covers about 5% of a child's visual function.

This book is an attempt to share information that will enable you to understand your child's problem better and point you in directions that will be helpful. It is beyond the scope of this book to provide specific tools and exercises in every case.

3. Anatomy of the Eye

The human eye is an anatomical masterpiece. The eye is about 24 mm in diameter and functions as the interface between the outside world and the inner world. The physical eye is responsible for capturing images from the outer world. It is similar to a video camera and, indeed, they have many things in common. However, the human eye is far superior to any camera built to date. For example, the human eye has much greater sensitivity to light. You can find your way in almost complete darkness as well as deal with bright sunlight on a beach. The video camera has a very limited range in comparison.

The eye muscles

There are six external muscles attached to each eye. These muscles work in pairs to enable you to move your eyes in all directions. Eye muscles are unique in their ability to move the eye very quickly and precisely to point it in the direction of what you want to observe. The muscles can also adjust in real time – for example, they allow you to track a tennis ball from one side of the court to the other.

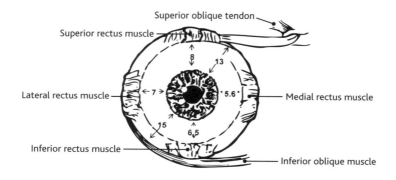

The four rectus muscles are located around the eye. The one above the eye (superior rectus) is the muscle responsible for moving the eye upward. The lower rectus muscle (inferior rectus) is responsible for moving the eye downward. These two muscles work in tandem to enable your eyes to move up and down to any degree. Horizontal movements of the eyes are performed by the medial rectus and lateral rectus muscles located on each side of the eye. These muscles move the eyes across the horizontal line. Together, the four rectus muscles give the eye the capacity to move in all directions.

In addition, there is also a pair of muscles attached to the back of the eye. These are called the oblique muscles because they allow the eyes to move both toward and away from each other. This enables you to point your eyes as well as track objects moving toward and away from you. The upper muscle (superior oblique) is attached to the bone near the nose with a long tendon. This muscle is used when you cross your eyes toward your nose.

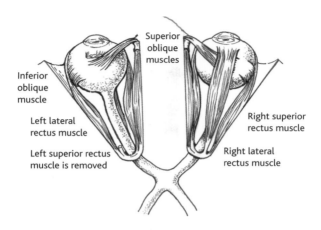

Your exterior eye muscles are also involved in adjusting the focus. In his pioneering research, William Bates, M.D. (1915) concluded that the oblique muscles focus by squeezing the eyeball and moving the retina into a position where the image is in perfect focus. He likened the function to that of a camera: when you want to focus it on something close-up, you move the lens forward. In the human eye the same principle is employed by squeezing the eyeball slightly to keep the image focused.

This action is mainly accomplished by the two oblique muscles. In myopia (near-sight), the back of the eye is permanently pushed out causing difficulty in focusing. With hyperopia (far-sight), the four rectus muscles are held very tightly causing the eyeball to become shorter. To give you an idea of the scale of these movements, each millimeter the eyeball is elongated is equivalent to approximately 3 diopters of myopia. With this degree of myopia, your vision would go from normal to being able to see clearly only up to 30 cm, approximately the normal reading distance. The physical changes that take place are minute, but they have huge consequences.

Inside the eye there are two circular muscles. One muscle determines the size of the iris and how much light enters the eye. The other muscle is circular in shape and is located around the lens.

The cornea

The clear part of the eye, the cornea, is responsible for about 75% of the focusing power of the eye. The greatest refractive effect is achieved at the interface between air and the tear film. This is why refractive surgery is possible. Shaving off even minute portions of the cornea has a major effect on the focusing power of the eye.

The cornea is about 0.5 mm thick at the center of the pupil and consists of several layers. The outer layer is the tear film, which nourishes the cornea as well as being part of the refractive element of the eye. You have probably noticed that blinking your eyes improves your ability to see. The physical surface of the cornea is called the epithelium, which consists of a protective layer of relatively hard surface cells. Their function is to protect the eye from damage. Extended wearing of contact lenses, especially hard lenses, eventually wears down the corneal epithelium and contact lenses can no longer be worn.

Just a few cells below the surface we have Bowman's layer. This is a layer of collagen-like cells that help the cornea to keep its shape – it is like the stiffeners in your shirt collar. This never heals if there has been a surgical intervention. The largest part of the cornea is the stroma. This is where laser surgery is performed: part of the stroma layer is blasted away, thinning the cornea so that the refractive power alters. Since there are no blood vessels in the cornea, it takes as much as six months to heal from surgery. It also leads to unavoidable weakening of the cornea.

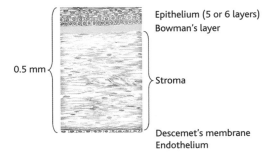

0.5 mm

Epithelium (5 or 6 layers)
Bowman's layer

Stroma

Descemet's membrane
Endothelium

Optical dimensions of the eye

This section is for those of you who are interested in the scientific aspects of the eye's optical dimensions. I am amazed that the eye is so small and that there are such huge differences in dioptric power between the cornea and the lens.

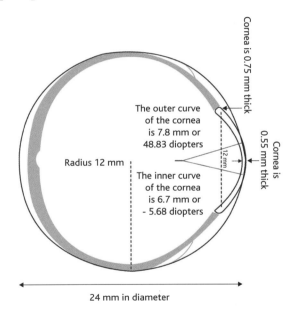

The lens

While the cornea provides most of the optical power of the eye, the lens is an important part of the optical system. The lens is about 10 mm in diameter and consists of crystalline cells that are completely transparent so light can shine through them.

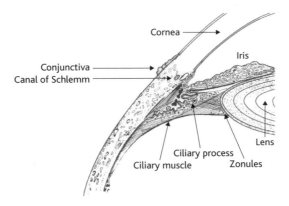

The lens is suspended in space by tiny fibers called zonules. Because of its high water content, the lens is very flexible and the pull of the zonules alters the shape of the lens. When the ciliary ring muscle is relaxed, the zonules are tightened and the lens becomes flatter, thus decreasing its focusing power. When the ciliary muscle is contracted, the zonules are relaxed and the lens bulges out, thus increasing its focal power. When the ciliary muscle is relaxed the eye is said to have "accommodated."

In vision tests, the drug atropine is sometimes used to paralyze the ciliary muscle. The rationale is that when ciliary muscle activity is eliminated you will get the "true" visual status. Some optometrists believe that this is the only valid test. Applying the same logic, you might wonder why your spine is not paralyzed when its height is measured to eliminate the possibility that you will stretch up and become taller!

The crystalline cells of the lens remain the same throughout our lives. Each year a new layer grows, like an onion. Between the ages of 20 and 80 the lens will have doubled in thickness. The lens has no blood vessels and it is nourished only by the aqueous humor which is continuously secreted from the ciliary body. Vitamin C is the most important supplement for the lens. The lens has the highest concentration of vitamin C in the entire body. Oxidation damage by free radicals can cause the crystalline cells to become opaque – a condition known as cataracts. Since the lens is only a small part of the optical system of the eye, you can still see even if your lens has been removed. Such a loss will amount to approximately 10% loss of visual acuity (or two lines on the eye-chart). Therefore, you could still be driving legally even without lenses in your eyes. The legal limit for driving is 20/40 visual acuity.

The retina

The retina is a paper-thin layer at the back of the eye which contains light-sensitive cells. If the retina is damaged then there will be permanent loss of vision. The most serious retina problems are macular degeneration and diabetic retinopathy, both of which are a form of deterioration of the integrity of the retina. Another problem is retinal detachment, which occurs in people with a high degree of myopia.

Photosensitive cells

There are two kinds of photosensitive cells in the eyes: rod cells, which operate under dim light conditions (referred to as scotopic vision) and cone cells, which give you sharp vision and color perception.

Rod cells are the most numerous – there are about 120 million. They are highly sensitive to low light and motion. Rod cells do not detect color and their visual acuity is about 20/200. Cone cells are used for sharp focus and color perception. The cone cells are concentrated in the central fovea located directly behind the iris and the other optical parts of the eye. Cone cell perception is referred to as photopic vision.

There are three types of cone cell, each sensitive to a specific range of light frequencies. The photo-pigment erythrolabe is sensitive to long-wave red light, chlorolabe is sensitive to mid-range green light and cyanolabe is sensitive to short-wave blue light. The three primary colors, red, green and blue, enable you to see all the colors in the spectrum. Blending the three basic colors can produce every hue imaginable. There are about 6,000,000 cone cells in each eye, with the highest density situated in the central fovea. Interestingly, there are no blue sensitive cone cells in the fovea. Their peak density lies just outside the central fovea. This accounts for the inability to see very small blue objects when they are centrally fixated.

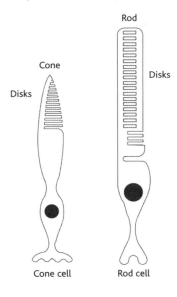

Rod cells contain the photosensitive pigment rhodopsin or visual purple. Named after its appearance, the rod cell consists of about 1,000 tiny disks, each one holding about 10,000 molecules of rhodopsin. Each molecule is capable of capturing one photon of light. The huge number of rhodopsin molecules means there is tremendous capacity for capturing light. When light falls on a rod cell, the rhodopsin becomes bleached. Only one quanta of light (the minimum amount of energy that can be carried in an electromagnetic wave) is required to bleach a molecule of rhodopsin. In fact, the scotopic spectral sensitivity of the eye corresponds to the properties of rhodopsin.

The macula

The retina has a central area, directly behind the cornea and lens, called the macula. At the center of the macula is the fovea. Vision and color perception are perfectly clear in this part of the eye. In the fovea, the photoreceptors have the densest concentration of light-sensitive cone cells, approximately 150,000 per square millimeter. These cells are also connected to a very large area of the visual cortex, which enables us to see clearly.

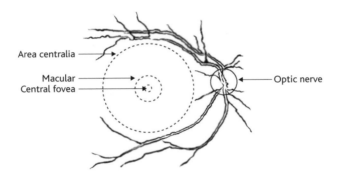

The macula is covered with a yellow pigment consisting of the carotenoids lutein and zeaxanthin. Traditionally it was believed that the yellow pigment aided visual resolution by filtering out the shorter blue light wavelength. This filtration effect is now considered to be a protection against blue light damage and, indirectly, a way of squelching free radical oxidation. Incidentally, the distribution of zeaxanthin seems to parallel that of cone cell photoreceptors.

The best dietary sources of carotenoids are dark-green leafy vegetables and yellow and red fruits. Carrots are the best source of beta-carotene and tomatoes supply lycopene. Zeaxanthin is the dominant carotenoid in vegetables such as orange peppers and sweetcorn, while most other vegetables, such as cabbage, spinach and watercress, are rich in lutein and beta-carotene.

4. Visual Development

The development of the visual system is partly "hard wired" and follows molecular cues. Other parts of the system develop from spontaneous visual stimuli. This means that the visual experiences of very young children influence their neural structures.

This reliance on optical experience can make the visual system vulnerable; if the environment is less than optimal, problems may develop. For instance, if children spend a lot of time involved in near-type visual activities, like playing video games, reading and schoolwork, we can end up with a predominantly near-sighted population. This is evident in some Asian countries, where up to 80% of high school students are near-sighted. In Singapore, 20% of 7-year-olds are near-sighted and 70% of college students are near-sighted (Seet et al., 2001). The Taiwan Health Ministry published a survey in 2006 showing that 85% of children at age 17 had near-sight.[1]

At birth most children are far-sighted by +2 to +3 diopters. Through a process called emmetropization, the eye undergoes a change in shape and size to become emmetropic (vision

---

1   See http://www.hpa.gov.tw/English/ClassPrint.aspx?No=201401160001/.

becoming normal) at around the age of 10. So, by this age the child should have perfect vision. If this development is disturbed, the eyeball may become too long (myopia, or near-sight) or too short (hyperopia, or far-sight).

At birth the eyeball is about 17 mm in diameter and grows about 0.016 mm a week. This growth mostly involves the back of the eyeball becoming longer. The lens inside the eye also increases in diameter. The eye grows about 1 mm every year until age 5, when the eyeball reaches around 21 mm in depth. The growth then slows down. At age 13, the eye has reached its full adult size of 24 mm. Children's eyes are especially sensitive to their visual environment from the ages of 6 to 14. In this period there is a tendency toward the rapid progression of myopia.

After birth the retina also continues to grow. The fovea, the point of absolutely clear vision, is fully developed at about 15 months. Stereopsis, or 3D vision, requires the brain to point both foveae at the same point in space. The eye movements must be perfectly co-ordinated to retain this relationship as the child moves their eyes around. Stereopsis is fully developed at about 24 months when it approaches adult levels.

Motion information is critical to many visual and motor functions – for example, perception of depth, estimating trajectories, isolating figures from the background, controlling posture and eye movements. The ability to recognize opposing directions of motion develops at about 10 to 13 weeks.

Emmetropization

The body always tries to find a perfect balance. The medical term for this is homeostasis. For example, if a liver from a small dog is implanted into a large dog, the liver will grow to fit the larger dog. The body knows when to start growing and when to stop growing. With regard to the eyes, this process is called emmetropization. Emmetropia is the term for perfect eyesight. Emmetropization is the process of the eyesight normalizing from being far-sighted at birth to becoming perfectly clear later on.

As mentioned above, this process can be impeded if the child's visual input is not what nature expected. For example, wearing glasses will cause the eyeball to change its growth pattern. The emmetropic balancing process is not controlled by genetics but by what the child sees – it is the visual environment that controls the process. When a child inhabits an environment that is predominantly near and close, the eyes experience hyperopic blur, which can lead to near-sight.

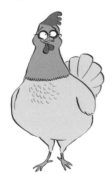

Schaeffel et al. (1988) did a pioneering study to find out what happens to visual development if you wear glasses. They used chicks because their eyes respond very quickly to external influences. The study revealed that wearing plus lenses caused the eyes to become more hyperopic, or far-sighted. Wearing minus lenses made the eyes become near-sighted. Schaeffel and his colleagues observe in their comments that with negative lenses the focal point is behind the retina, which induces a strong tendency for the eyeball to lengthen. With positive lenses, the sharp image is in front of the retina, which stunts the growth of the eye. Apparently the eye grows toward the optimum sharpness of the image. If they fitted a plus lens in one eye and a minus lens on the other, the same thing happened. Of course, the control chicks' eyes did not actually change. This study has since been replicated many times with various animals with the same or similar results.

Later, Schaeffel and his colleagues found that if only half of the eye is covered with a lens, then only that half alters its growth while the other side remains the same (Schaeffel et al., 1988). This proves that the eye does respond to the visual environment. This is still partly true even if the optic nerve to the brain has been severed. The eye has an inbuilt intelligence which controls its growth, in addition to the mechanism in the brain which also controls the development of the eye.

Of course, chick eyes and human eyes are very different, so how about studies with animals that have eyes more like human eyes? One such study, done by Smith (1998), set out to determine whether early development of the eyes was regulated by visual feedback.

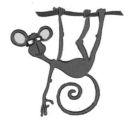

Smith wanted to find out if infant monkeys could compensate for vision altering lenses. The study showed that when lenses of different powers were used for the left and right eye, the axes of both eyes grew to different lengths. In this way, the refractive imbalance between the two eyes was reduced. When the monkeys were fitted with equally powered lenses in both eyes, the growth of the eyeball was modified. For lenses between -3 and +6 diopters, the changes were primarily due to growth in the axial length – that is, the eyeball altered its development to compensate for the lens. Limiting growth was observed with plus lenses and increasing growth with minus lenses. When the lenses were removed, the monkeys had an unrestricted visual experience. The eyeballs consistently grew toward emmetropia, or normal clear vision.

Smith concluded that spectacles worn in early life can predictably alter the ocular growth and refractive status of one or both eyes by changing the eye's effective focus. This raises the following question: if lenses can predictably alter growth in the eyeball of a monkey, does it follow that it would be possible to use lenses to prevent myopia from developing?

At City College in New York, Zhu and colleagues (2003) conducted a study using chicks to determine whether brief periods of positive lens wear could outweigh day-long wearing of negative lenses. They found that wearing positive lenses for as little as 12 minutes (six intervals of two minutes) a day, with vision unrestricted during the remainder of the time, caused the eyes to become hyperopic and reduced the rate of ocular elongation. This held true even when the chicks wore negative lenses for entire days, except for eight minutes wearing positive lenses. The eye compensated for the positive lens as if the negative lens had not been worn. In their conclusion, the researchers state: "if the hyperopic defocus of long daily periods of reading predisposes a child to myopia, then regular, brief interruptions of reading might have use as a prophylaxis against progression of myopia."

Over one hundred years of study brings us to the same conclusion: overuse of the eyes during near work is the main cause of myopia.

5. Visual Skill Development

Vision skills are learned. As a child grows, these skills are assembled, like toy building blocks, and are naturally developed one after the other. Many of the games children play are actually developing their vision skills. The foundation skills for reading are built years before the child is ready to actually learn to read.

In some children, the basic skills are not fully mastered and they will have difficulties. Exactly what causes the difficulty may not be apparent without proper testing. However, most of these problems are not solved by fitting glasses. It is a matter of development, so it can be trained – just like any skill can be improved through practice.

I have described below the normal stages of vision development and how parents can promote this development.

Infant – the first four months

Newborn babies can see patterns of light and dark as well as shades of gray. Initially, newborns can only focus about 25 cm – just enough to see mommy's face. Infants soon begin to follow moving objects with their eyes, and tracking and eye co-ordination start to develop. They also begin to reach for objects and develop their eye–hand co-ordination. At 4 months babies can also see colors.

4 to 6 months

At this age, babies learn to push themselves up, roll over, sit and scoot. Eye and body co-ordination development continues as they learn how to control their own movements in space. At 4 to 6 months, babies become quite skillful with their eye–hand co-ordination and are able to grasp toys freely or direct a bottle to their mouth.

By the fourth month, babies have finished learning how to fuse the images coming from each eye into a complete three-dimensional image. There is now spatial and dimensional awareness when reaching for an object. Babies continue to refine their eye co-ordination and focusing skills. They learn how to quickly and accurately shift between near and far objects. A child's normal vision, or 20/20, has usually developed at about 6 months when they begin to babble.

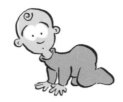

6 to 8 months

Most children start to crawl at this time, further developing their eye–body co-ordination. At this age, babies also discover how to set visual goals – seeing something and moving toward it. This is a time of great exploration and many new experiences. There is rapid development of visual perception skills as the baby experiences their own body in relation to other objects and they begin to notice differences in size, shape and position. At 8 months babies have developed fairly accurate eye movements.

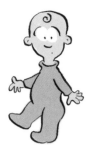

8 to 12 months

At this age, babies now can judge distance well. Eye–hand co-ordination allows them to throw toys fairly accurately. Perception skills, such as visual memory, visual discrimination and the ability to determine exact characteristics and distinctive features among similar objects or forms, help babies make sense of their world. Vision and fine motor movements are now sufficiently well-developed that they can manipulate small objects. They can begin to feed themselves with finger foods. Once children start walking, they learn how to use their eyes to direct and co-ordinate their body movements. At 12 months babies begin to say "Mama" and "Dada."

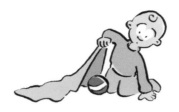

Pre-school

Children's vision continues to develop. As toddlers, it is important for them to maintain the development of eye–hand and eye–body co-ordination with games such as stacking and assembling toy building blocks, rolling balls, coloring, drawing and cutting out. It is also important to read to children to develop their visualization skills as they can begin to picture the story in their minds. When you are reading to your child, take his or her finger and run it across the words you are reading. Encourage them to practice drawing horizontal lines, always moving from left to right, as this develops correct eye movements for reading later on. Drawing a continuous horizontal line is a sign of good left–right laterality development.

Ask your child to cut out shapes, beginning with a square and a circle. This activity develops their ability to recognize shapes and forms an important skill which is needed to learn the alphabet. Together with the child, discover round and square patterns all over the place. Then start sorting them out by looking for similarities and differences – for example, the child can help to put away the cutlery after washing up – the spoons go here, the forks go here and so on. Sorting toys into different categories is also great practice.

This is also a good time to start to teach your child basic math concepts. Start with counting up to at least ten. Counting develops the visual and auditory memory and sequencing skills. The child also needs to have a concept of what the numbers mean. A wonderful way of teaching this is to use beads or buttons so they can actually *see* what five or ten looks like.

When appropriate, include the idea that you can add beads/ buttons to get a bigger number or you can subtract so you end up with fewer beads/buttons. Introduce comparison words like *more*, *bigger*, *less* and *take away*. Always use concrete words so the child can build up visual images of what the words mean.

When the child understands the concept of counting you can introduce measurement. The amount a vessel can hold, such as full, empty or half full, needs to be seen before the child will begin to understand these ideas. Next come the concepts of length and height. Compare the child's toys, perhaps sorting them according to height or length. Again, it is important that the child experiences these concepts using all of their senses – that is seeing, feeling, naming and talking about the differences.

Time is another abstract concept that can be introduced. Together with time comes words like *before*, *after*, *early* and *late* to understand what happens first and last. This concept can be illustrated when you bake a cake. Assemble all the ingredients and lay them out in the order you are going to use them so the child can visualize the sequence of events.

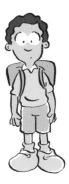

Schoolchildren

As young children grow up they spend more or less equivalent time looking at things close and far away, so they are using all their visual skills in equal measure. School, on the other hand, requires children's eyes to focus on close work for extended periods every day. As they progress in their academic learning, there is more and more emphasis on reading and close work. In some cases this can lead to vision problems, such as near-sight (myopia); others develop far-sight which may lead to eyestrain. Poor eye co-ordination is another cause of reading problems.

Therefore it is important to preserve children's natural clear vision and introduce Vision Training exercises when appropriate, to bring back the natural vision. Remember, clear eyesight is a birth right.

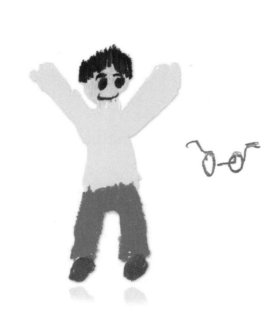

6. Visual Efficiency Skills

Smooth and well co-ordinated eye movements are an important basis for good visual efficiency. All movement of the eyes is done by the six external eye muscles (see Chapter 3). Four of them are located in front of the eye – one on top and one on the bottom and one on each side of the eye. There are two other muscles located at the back of the eye. These muscles enable you to rotate your eyes in and out, as you do when reading. All of these movements are controlled by the brain. Visual efficiency determines how well you see near and far, as well as how well your eyes work together.

Visual acuity – how well you see, close-up as well as at a distance – is referred to as focusing or accommodation. Problems with visual acuity are called refractive errors. This is the skill that is tested when you go to the optometrist for an eye test.

If you have difficulty seeing objects in the distance you are myopic, or near-sighted. This is the most common problem. If you have difficulty seeing close-up you are hyperopic, or far-sighted. This may cause eyestrain when reading. Fortunately, both respond very well to Vision Training.

Metric system

Snellen

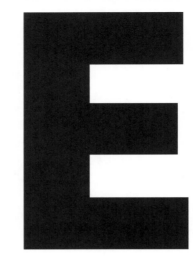

6/133

20/400

E

6/120

20/200

KR

6/48

20/160

LVD

6/3.5

20/125

ZSHC

Metric system		Snellen
6/24	**CHGKRN**	20/80
6/21	**DCNRSPKE**	20/70
6/18	**HONGSDCV**	20/60
6/15	**OKHGDTNVRCS**	20/50
6/12	**YOUCANDRIVENOW**	20/40
6/7.5	**BDCLKZVHSROA**	20/30
6/6.75	**HKGBCANOMPVESR**	20/25
6/6	**YOUHAVEPERFECTEYESIGHT**	20/20
6/4.6	**THISISEVENBETTERYOUHAVEMAGICEYES**	20/16

Snellen chart

Designed for viewing at 3 meters. Letter size and distance is important for accurate measurement.
Please download this chart from www.vision-training.com/en/Download/Download.html

Also note that many medications negatively affect the visual system. Common medications that influence the ability to focus include antihistamines, phenytoin (used to treat epilepsy), methylphenidate (e.g. Ritalin) and dextroamphetamine (e.g. Dexedrine) (both used to treat attention-deficit disorder (ADD) and attention-deficit hyperactivity disorder (ADHD)).

The vision test

Visual acuity is tested using eye-charts, a retinoscopy or an autorefractor. On the familiar Snellen chart, you should be able to see 8.278 mm letters at a distance of 20 feet (6 meters). Children can normally see 20/16 or better than 20/20. Thus a 10-year-old can easily read the bottom line of the eye-chart.

A 10-year-old can also see objects clearly as close as 5 cm and read text that is printed in 3 point font. A child with normal near vision can read this print in daylight from about 8 cm from his or her eyes.

Here is the same paragraph in 3 point font:

A 10-year-old can also see objects clearly as close as 5 cm and read text that is printed in 3 point font. A child with normal near vision can read this print in daylight from about 8 cm from his or her eyes.

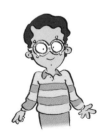

If the child can't see the third line on the eye-chart, a subjective trial-and-error test is done by trying out lenses of various power until the ophthalmologist finds a lens that is effective and comfortable. This test is based on the child's feedback, thus the subjective nature. The lens power should start from 0 (plano) and gradually increase until the child gets clear vision. If the subjective test starts at the child's previous prescription you tend to get glasses that are too strong. The child adapts to the stronger and stronger lenses as the test progresses.

Experienced optometrists often start with a retinoscopy. This is actually the most accurate test available. It consists of shining a light into the child's eyes. The optometrist can then see whether the child is near-sighted or far-sighted. After the other tests are done, they verify the reading a second time with the retinoscope.

For Vision Training purposes, we then lower the lens power by 10–15% so the eyes have room to improve. Remember, the eyes have to adjust to the lens power. If the lenses are too powerful, the child's vision will be adversely impacted – that is, their eyesight will deteriorate.

How to check if your child's glasses are too powerful

A simple way for you to check if your child's glasses are too strong is to ask them to stand at the 3 meter mark (for eye-charts designed for 3 meters) wearing his or her glasses. If the child can see the second line then the glasses are 100% corrected and will limit the child's ability to improve his or her eyesight. It is time to get lenses with lower power.

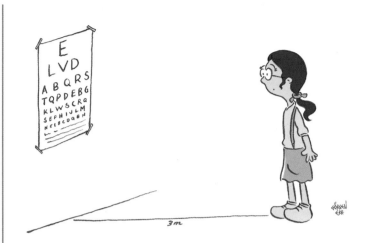

The new glasses should correct the child's vision just enough so that they can read the fourth line (the 20/30). It does not have to be clear as long as the letters are readable. This is about 10% lower and it is legal for driving. These glasses will not impair the child at school, such as the ability to read the board in the classroom. I do not recommend that you reduce the lens power beyond 20/40, or the fifth line from the bottom on the eye-chart. If you do this, then the child will have to strain to see and do schoolwork.

Of course, the next best step is to do Vision Training exercises and restore the child's vision back to normal.

-2 diopters or less

With a prescription of -2 diopters a child can see clearly out to 50 cm, so there is no need for them to wear their glasses for reading or other near work. However, they will need glasses when copying from the board at school. But remember, the damaging effect on the child's eyes can be substantial if they wear glasses all the time.

-4 diopters or more

Fortunately, prescriptions of -4 diopters are less common. A child with strong minus lenses will need to wear a special pair of glasses for reading with a lower lens power. When reading we naturally change -3 diopters. So, if a child wears -4 diopters then they will actually have to change by -7 diopters (-3 + -4 = -7 diopters). So, if they do a fair amount of reading, this will cause the visual system to adapt toward -7 diopters – in other words, slowly getting worse.

Therefore, it is better to have a pair of lower power glasses specifically for reading, as these will be less damaging. This same recommendation applies for adults.

Visual acuity

A visual efficiency test may uncover the following acuity problems:

- Myopia (near-sight)
- Hyperopia (far-sight)
- Anisometropia (a difference between the eyes)
- Astigmatism (uneven muscle tension pattern)

Accommodative disorders or focusing problems

A test may also reveal the following physical problems:

- Accommodative insufficiency
- Accommodative excess
- Accommodative infacility
- Presbyopia (this condition is associated with ageing so doesn't affect children)

Binocular vision disorders (problems with both eyes)

Strabismus

- Esotropia (one eye turns in)
- Exotropia (one eye turns out)
- Hypertropia (one eye turns up)
- Hypotropia (one eye turns down)

Phorias (double vision)

- Esophoria (inward deviation of the eye)
- Exophoria (outward deviation of the eye)
- Hyperphoria (upward deviation of the eye)
- Hypophoria (downward deviation of the eye)

Amblyopia (lazy eye)

- Strabismic amblyopia (due to strabismus)
- Anisometropic amblyopia (due to differences between the eyes)

- Isometropic amblyopia (in both eyes resulting from large, approximately equal, uncorrected refractive errors, namely hyperopia, of more than 5 diopters, and myopia, of more than 10 diopters)

- Stimulus deprivation amblyopia (when the eye has been closed for extended periods of time – this may happen if eye patches are worn for too long)

- Hysterical amblyopia (when psychological factors are involved)

Ocular mobility disorders (eye movements especially related to reading)

- Saccadic dysfunction
- Pursuit dysfunction
- Fixation disorder

7. Focusing Efficiency

At birth focusing is poorly developed. A newborn is able to focus to about 30 cm from their eyes – just enough to see mom or dad's face. During the first three months, depth of focus decreases and the focusing response improves. The primary trigger for focusing to activate is blur: the things you want to see are unclear so the focusing mechanism is activated. Through the first six months there is a rapid development, so the focusing ability is fully developed in a 6-month-old baby.

Behavioral optometrists believe that children with reading difficulties have a high rate of focusing disorders due to accommodative infacility. Hoffman (1986) examined 107 learning disabled children in whom he found very high degrees of binocular or eye co-ordination problems (87%). Accommodative or focusing problems were found in 83% of the children. Hoffman also found that almost all of them (95%) had ocular mobility or eye movement issues which interfered with their ability to read. There appears to be ample evidence for the behavioral optometrist's claim.

Children must be able to sustain the average eye-to-desk distance of 30 cm (3 diopter focusing or accommodative demand) for 30–45 minutes or longer. If they are lacking in sufficient visual power or stamina, the child will develop visual fatigue or will resort to avoidance behaviors. This will be particularly true for far-sighted children, since they need to use more power to focus their eyes on the book. Without the required visual stamina to focus for the duration they simply get tired.

Modern ergonomically designed school desks are adjustable so the proper reading distances can be altered with the natural growth of the child. These desks also have a book rest that is further away than is traditional – a recognition that many first graders are far-sighted. It would also be helpful if books could be printed with larger lettering, so that it is easier for the child to read without straining their focusing system.

Behavioral cues to look out for, especially after a long period of reading or near work, include:

- Reports blurry vision at near tasks.

- Reports blurry vision at a distance after near work.

- Reports eye fatigue after short periods of reading or writing.

- Holds book too close.

- Has difficulty sustaining near tasks.

- Rubs eyes excessively.

- Reports feeling a pulling sensation around the eyes.

- Has red eyes.

● Is tired and sleepy.

● Avoids near-vision tasks like reading.

If you observe any of these symptoms, especially blurry distance vision after reading, then it is advisable to investigate further.

There are three main focusing problems. These have different causes but very similar effects.

1. Accommodative insufficiency

If a child has accommodative insufficiency then the amount of focusing ability available (the amplitude of accommodation) is less than what is expected for their age. The child will experience intermittent blurred vision when reading. In an attempt to obtain clear vision, they will try harder and this may lead to some of the symptoms listed above.

2. Accommodative excess

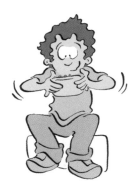

Accommodative excess occurs when the child is overdoing reading or playing video games. They will have blurred vision when looking away from the book or games device. This may also lead to myopia. Initially this myopia is referred to as pseudomyopia (temporary myopia) or, putting it simply, tired eyes. If the

45

activity is continued it becomes real myopia and the child is fitted with minus glasses. In Asia, pseudomyopia is the leading cause of myopia and increasingly so in other parts of the world as more children spend hours every day on computers or video games. It is interesting to note that pseudomyopia can also be induced by wearing the wrong glasses.

3. Accommodative infacility

This is a condition in which the amplitude of accommodation, or visual power, is normal but the speed of the response is reduced. The most common complaint with accommodative infacility is blurred vision when looking from near to far and back again. The child will find that it takes a while before their vision is clear.

Testing focusing efficiency

Most optometrists and eye doctors only test the amplitude of accommodation. However, only presbyopia and accommodative insufficiency can be detected using this method. The child should also be tested for accommodative facility. This tests their ability to change focus rapidly near and far for a sustained period of time. It is the only suitable method for detecting accommodative infacility. Obviously, this is a key test because it will reveal the actual problem the child is experiencing.

The optometrist may test for both negative relative accommodation (NRA) and positive relative accommodation (PRA). NRA is a measure of the maximum ability to relax accommodation with clear vision, and PRA measures the maximum ability to accommodate.

The test is as follows: after the distance correction is established, the child is instructed to look at small letters at reading distance. The optometrist now adds lenses in -0.25 diopter increments until they report that the text has become blurry. The total value of the minus lenses added is the positive relative accommodation. Values over -3.50 diopters will indicate accommodative excess, or over-worked eyes. Children with accommodative insufficiency typically have values less than -1.50 diopters.

The standard method for testing accommodative facility is a lens rocking procedure using a pair of +2 diopter lenses on one side of a flipper and -2 diopters on the other side. The test is done at normal reading distance. The child starts off by trying to read through the -2 diopter lens. When they report that the text has become clear, the lenses are flipped to +2 diopters. Again, when the child reports that the text is clear, the lens is flipped again. This flipping is done for one minute. The optometrist counts the number of cycles (changes). Assuming there are no eye co-ordination issues, the child should be able to do eight cycles per minute using both eyes.

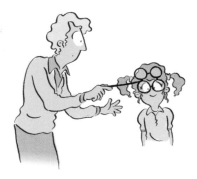

Another important way of evaluating the child's focusing ability is near-point retinoscopy. This is particularly useful in detecting accommodative excess. A dynamic retinoscopy technique called monocular estimate method (MEM) is a reliable measure of accommodative accuracy (i.e. lag and response). MEM is carried out under normal reading conditions, including reading distance, angle of view, posture and lighting. In other words, the actual environment in which the child is

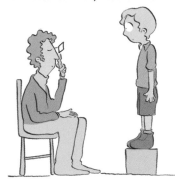

reading is approximated for the test. This is because it is important to rule out all possible factors that might influence the accuracy of the test.

For the test, the child is asked to read words on a card that is attached to the retinoscope. The optometrist interposes plus lenses with varying power in-between the retinoscope and the eye until the lag of accommodation is neutralized. The lens is interposed only briefly, so there is minimal interference with the natural focusing response.

The normal range of accommodative lag expected for children aged between 5 and 12 years is from plano (no power) to +0.75 diopters. If the lag is more than +0.75 diopters the child may be far-sighted. Of course, the influence of prescription medications and so on must be ruled out. A 10-year-old has a maximum of about 12.50 diopters of accommodative amplitude. Falling 2 diopters below this is usually associated with symptoms such as far-sightedness. Hofstetter's formula for predicting the minimum range of accommodative amplitude at different ages is:

$$D = 15 - \text{one quarter of the child's age}$$

So, for a 9-year-old, the minimum expected amplitude is 12.75 diopters (15 − 2.25).

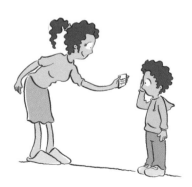

Testing amplitude of accommodation

Reliable evaluation of a child's accommodative facility can be carried out from the age of 7. To test the focusing power of your child's eyes, you need a tape measure and a small card printed with text at a 14 point font size, like this:

CAPITAL LETTERS ARE EASIER.

To perform the test, follow these instructions:

1. Ask the child to cover one eye.

2. Hold the card about 3 cm from the eye and slowly move it out until the child says the text is clear.

3. Measure the distance from the eye to the near point of clear focus.

4. To get the amplitude of accommodation divide 100 by the measurement you have taken.

   (e.g. if the near point is 8 cm then the amplitude of accommodation is 100 divided by 8 = 12.50)

5. Compare the amplitude with what is expected at that age (use Hofstetter's formula above). The minimum expected amplitude is 15 diopters minus a quarter of the child's age. If the amplitude of accommodation works out to more than 2 diopters less than what is expected, further tests will be necessary.

Years of age	Diopters
7	13.25
8	13.00
9	12.75
10	12.50
11	12.25
12	12.00

Amplitude of accommodation

Training accommodative amplitude

Here is a simple way to develop your child's focusing stamina. Have the child look at one spot, a flower perhaps, at a distance. They should have one arm straight out with their thumb pointing up. Tell them to hold the other thumb as close as possible, yet still clear in sight.

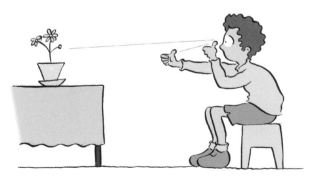

Ask the child to first look at the closest thumb, then jump to the thumb at arm's length and finally to the flower at a distance. A child with perfect accommodative amplitude can do this easily. If the flower is blurry or double then continue the exercise until the skill improves. Perhaps start with the flower at a closer distance to make it easier for the child.

Note: The near point, where the thumb is clear as close as possible, should be less than 12 cm from the eye. If the near point is further out than this, then this indicates a problem. In some countries, such as Taiwan, doctors recommend applying atropine drops every night in an attempt to slow down the development of myopia. Unfortunately, however, this causes the near point of clear vision to move further outward as well as producing undesirable symptoms. The same is the case if the child wears strong plus lenses for hyperopia. (See Chapter 14 for how to deal with hyperopia.)

8. Eye Movement Skills

Ocular mobility refers to how well you move your eyes. This is the skill that allows you to accurately jump your eyes from one object to another (saccades) and to track moving objects (pursuit) – like following a particular car on a busy street. The ability to fixate on a particular object allows you to keep it in focus briefly, as when you are reading and your eyes jump from one word group to another at the rate at which you integrate the information. Smooth and accurate eye movements are very important when it comes to paying attention, reading properly and doing well in sports.

If there is a difference between the eyes – for example, if one eye is weaker than the other – then you need to balance the vision (see the exercises in Chapter 16). Imbalance (anisometropia) can also make reading more difficult.

Eye movement assessment involves checking fixation maintenance, pursuit and saccadic eye movements. Fixation maintenance represents the ability to maintain a steady image on the retina. We do this when we are reading. Good readers use a stepping movement of the eyes as they fixate on one word or a group of words on the line they are reading. If you have problems with fixation, then you may not be aware that you are jumping up a line from the one you want to read, or you may be randomly dropping down a line. You may also drop or lose two- or three-letter words along the way (e.g. and, the, two, me, he, she).

Pursuit eye movements represent the ability to remain fixed on a moving target and ignore the background. This is a vital skill if you want to participate in any team sport, such as football, handball, hockey and so on. To be good at these sports you need to know where your team mates are and to predict where they will be next. If you don't quite know where they are, you are not likely to be on the team for long!

These two eye movement skills are vital when it comes to reading. Research shows that up to 85% of children who have reading difficulties lack efficiency in one or both skills (see Rosner and Gruber, 1985).

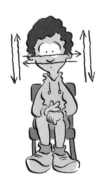 The optometrist or eye doctor may test eye movement by doing the "H" ocular movement test: using a pen or some small object and moving it in the shape of a "H" about 30 cm from the child's eyes. They will look at the child's eyes and judge if there are any areas where the eyes do not follow easily. You can also do this yourself.

Eye movement skills

Fixation – holding the image of a steady object focused on the retina (e.g. reading a word).

Vestibulo-ocular reflex – holding images of the seen world steady on the retina during brief head movements.

Optokinetic reflex – holding images of the seen world steady during slow head movements (e.g. shifting the gaze from one side to another).

Smooth pursuit – holding the image of a moving object focused on the retina (e.g. when you are following a car on the road and ignoring the background).

Saccades – directing images of eccentrically located objects of interest onto the retina. This occurs when reading because the brain previews the words before they come into clear view.

Vergence – co-ordinating the eyes and moving them in and out, so that the image of a single object is placed simultaneously on the retina of both eyes and fused into one image.

However, the most effective way to test eye movement skills is with a Visagraph mask. This is an ingenious device which uses infrared sensors to accurately trace the movements of the eyes while reading. The equipment is connected to a computer

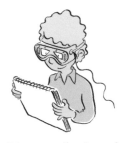

software package which analyzes and displays a graph of how the eyes move while the child is reading. This is by far the most accurate way of measuring what the eyes do while reading. For instance, the graphs reveal the number of fixations per 100 words and the time of fixation connected with the length of the word. The speed of reading is measured by words per minute and you can see at once which age level this corresponds to. You can also compare the movements of the left and right eye. In combination with Vision Training and a reading skill program, the Visagraph can also display any progress the child makes.

What is a Visagraph test?

The Visagraph was developed by Stanford E. Taylor. It is an ingenious eye movement recording device, incorporated into a pair of goggles, which is used to accurately capture what happens when a child is reading. This test is the gold standard when it comes to testing eye movement when reading.

The device records eye movements while the child reads ten lines of easy-to-read text. This data is then saved to software on an ordinary personal computer for analysis. A graph can be printed out that accurately shows how the eyes move. In addition, an animation is available that shows how the eyes move over the text. This is extremely useful since it shows the child what his or her eyes are doing. It can also be used to show progress if repeated after training.

The graph below is from a good reader. You can see the staircase pattern as the eye fixates on words along the line.

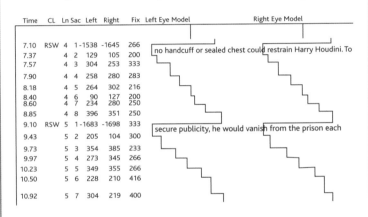

Time	CL	Ln	Sac	Left	Right	Fix	Left Eye Model / Right Eye Model
7.10	RSW	4	1	-1538	-1645	266	no handcuff or sealed chest could restrain Harry Houdini. To
7.37		4	2	129	105	200	
7.57		4	3	304	253	333	
7.90		4	4	258	280	283	
8.18		4	5	264	302	216	
8.40		4	6	90	127	200	
8.60		4	7	234	280	250	
8.85		4	8	396	351	250	
9.10	RSW	5	1	-1683	-1698	333	secure publicity, he would vanish from the prison each
9.43		5	2	205	104	300	
9.73		5	3	354	385	233	
9.97		5	4	273	345	266	
10.23		5	5	349	355	266	
10.50		5	6	228	210	416	
10.92		5	7	304	219	400	

This graph shows a child with poor eye movement skills. It is clear that the two eyes are not working together and there are frequent regressions.

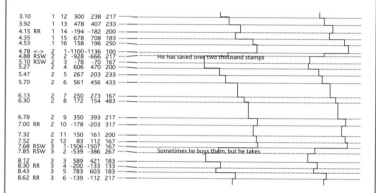

Taylor recommended that all children are tested with the Visagraph at 9 years, 12 years and 14 years to make sure that eye movements are well established and have become automatic. The test doesn't take long, so if your child has difficulty reading, look for an optometrist who uses the Visagraph. If your child's eyes are not working together properly, just looking from word to word will require a lot of effort.

A simpler way to approximate the Visagraph is to use a piece of string to check whether the eyes maintain their convergence point while reading.

Testing convergence

This test provides accurate feedback on whether the two eyes converge. When you view a string held on your nose and pulled out directly in front of you, you will see two strings forming an "X," "V" or "Y." The crossing point should be exactly where you place your finger or tie a knot. The convergence point should be exactly through the center of the knot, and it should remain steady when you move the string from side to side horizontally. If not, there is a convergence issue which may result in reading difficulties.

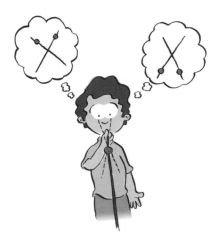

Here's how to do the test:

1. Tie a knot in a piece of string at the normal reading distance of about 30 cm (approximately the length from hand to hand stretched across your chest).

2. Ask the child to place one end of the string on their nose.

3. Position the knot roughly where the top of a page would be and slowly move it from left to right, as when reading. Move the knot down the imaginary page with a zig-zag movement.

4. Ask the child to tell you if the crossing point moves in or out as the knot travels the imaginary page.

5. If the crossing point moves in or out at any point, then there is a potential problem with pursuit skills.

Sometimes, as you move the string all the way to one side, you will notice the child's co-ordination gets lost. If your child is showing signs of pursuit problems, then encourage them to mentally control the position of the crossing point so it is always exactly on the knot.

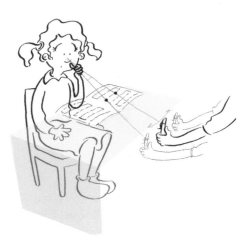

Testing for these skills is unfortunately something optometrists and eye doctors often omit in their standard testing procedures. However, if your child has problems in this area, it is a major issue because it gets worse as they get tired.

One gentleman in his sixties told me that since childhood he had only ever been able to read one word at a time. Imagine going through school like that! When we did the convergence test, we discovered that his crossing point moved in and out as his eyes traveled horizontally across the imaginary page. This meant that his eyes would lose focus as he moved from word to word; focusing either behind or above the page can cause the words to appear double or invisible. He was thrilled when he discovered that he could actually keep the crossing point on the knot all the way across and up and down the imaginary page.

Another example was a boy in Sydney, Australia. During lunch, he told me that he could not see what he was writing, he felt it. I watched him while he wrote, "The fox jumps over the fence." I noticed that his crossing point was actually about 8 cm above the paper on which he was writing. This is called convergence insufficiency and is present in many children diagnosed with attention-deficit hyperactivity disorder (ADHD) and dyslexia. (Try holding one of your fingers about 5 cm above the page as you read this. Look at your finger and continue reading. You will have experienced the convergence insufficiency this boy suffered when reading or writing. It is possible to read like this, but it is very strenuous and you become tired extremely quickly.) By the way, after lunch the boy's father was amazed that he was happily reading the Sunday newspaper magazine without his glasses!

Eye movement exercise

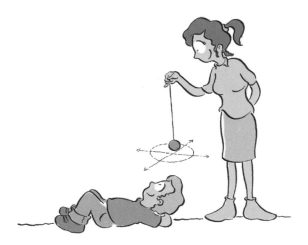

Here is a simple exercise that will help children to learn to move their eyes smoothly in all directions. You will need a brightly colored tennis ball, or similar, and some string.

1. Attach the string to the ball so you can move it around like a pendulum.

2. Ask the child to lie down on their back. Make sure that there is no light shining down directly into their eyes.

3. Stand behind the child's head so that you can move the ball out to about 50 cm over their eyes. Move the ball in patterns so that they can follow it with smooth eye movements. Move your body rather than swing the ball. Repeat each pattern three times. The exercise should take about three minutes in total.

Ideally, the eyes of an 8-year-old should move effortlessly. Younger children may not yet have this level of control. Look for skips, stickiness, stutter, darting ahead or backward or frozen stares. If you notice any of these symptoms, start by moving the ball slowly so the child can train their eye muscles to move in the direction that they find difficult. Repeating this exercise two or three times a day will lead to quick improvements. After a few days or weeks, the child will have developed the ability to move their eyes in fluid movements.

Testing saccadic movements

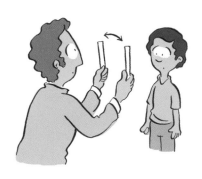

To test for saccadic (fast) eye movement in children above 7 years, hold two pencils (one red and one yellow) at about reading distance and a book width apart. Ask the child to look alternately at the red and the yellow pencil while you watch their eyes. Their eyes should switch rapidly and accurately from one pencil to the other. They should be able to do this rapidly five times without error.

Another way to test saccadic movements is the Developmental Eye Movement (DEM) test, which involves the child reading out differently spaced numbers. You can make your own eye movement test charts using a spreadsheet or word-processing software. Create the first page with two columns of 20 two-digit numbers, one in the left margin and the other in the right margin – an example can be found on page 66. Use this for testing the vertical saccades. Next, make a second page with five randomly spaced numbers across each line (but not more than 16 lines) – an example is on page 67. This is for testing the horizontal saccades.

Before starting the test, ask the child not to use his or her fingers when reading.

1. Get the child to hold the first page in their normal reading position.

2. Ask them to read out the numbers from the first column and then the second, carefully but as fast as possible.

3. Time the exercise and note where the child makes a mistake (there may be omissions, additions, substitutions or transpositions). Score by counting the number of errors.

4. Take the second sheet and ask the child to read it line by line as quickly as possible.

5.   Again, notice if there are mistakes or lines skipped. Add up the number of errors.

A normal reader should be able to do this without making any mistakes. If you notice more than three mistakes then you may need to investigate further. The best option is to get a Visagraph test done, which is much more accurate.

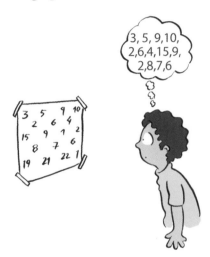

The second sheet can also serve as an exercise on its own. Repeat the test a few times and you may notice that the child can do it without making any mistakes. After a few days, repeat the exercise again. If the child can do it without making a mistake then they probably have no problem with saccadic eye movements.

12	20
16	48
75	99
14	63
22	49
56	76
35	37
21	63
92	11
24	62
51	83
93	16
13	49
65	71
33	49
16	22
17	66
29	30
49	50
88	19

Testing Saccadic movements – vertical

12		52			82	41					66
44			91			22			67		31
52	89			67			70				46
11		15		99				32			83
44			77			68				93	18
62				45			23		92		55
23		65	90			75					74
56				33			29			16	69
99	23		66					78			24
10		53			29		34				81
13			28			67			84		98
36		27			25			71			63
36			48			53				95	66
72	25			73			37				90
15		28			52				73		14
16			32				69			51	88

Testing Saccadic movements – horizontal

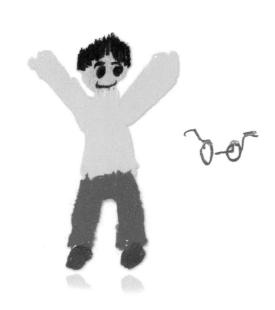

9. Evaluation of Phorias

Some children develop a problem known as exophoria, which is a tendency for the eyes to deviate in an outward direction. If it cannot be compensated for, this can cause double vision. This is different from (manifest) strabismus where you can actually see the eye turn outward (also known as exotropia).

If one or both eyes has a tendency to deviate outward, then the child must exert more effort in order to read with clear vision. Most studies show that the more effort a child has to use while reading, the lower their comprehension and reading performance. If exophoria exists, each time fixation is moved to the next word, the eyes will tend to deviate outward and must be brought back to retain clear focus. This may cause the eyes to slide a few letters outward, and the result may be reversed letters or words.

Testing for phorias

The simplest test for phorias, both near and far, is to use a Maddox rod. This is a piece of grooved plastic or glass which is created from a series of parallel convex cylinder lenses. Often it is colored red.

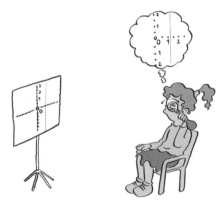

The optometrist holds a test card with a light at the center at reading distance. The child holds the Maddox rod in front of one eye and looks at the light. With normal eyes, a phantom red line will appear in the center through the light. However, if there is any phoria, the red line will be displaced either to the left or to the right of the light to the same degree in prism diopters of the phoria.

It is also possible to have vertical phoria, so the test can also be done to assess this problem. The Maddox rod is simply turned so that the lines are horizontal. The child will see the line as deviating upward or downward if there is any phoria present.

It is important that this test is done at the distance and angle at which the child usually reads, as well as at the distance of the classroom board. In this way, the test replicates as closely as possible the actual conditions the child will experience.

The optometrist will typically correct the phoria by adding a prism to the child's glasses to compensate for the deviation. However, this will only work at the one set distance. It does not address the underlying problem.

You can approximate the Maddox rod test by using the string test in Chapter 8. Check where the phantom cross appears at the child's reading angle and distance. Move the string left and right in the air, the knot approximating the location that a book would be positioned when the child is reading.

If the strings seem to move apart, the child has a phoria at that angle and distance. If the crossing point does not stay on the knot, and moves inward, there is a convergence insufficiency. If the crossing point moves out, the child has convergence excess. This should be trained away as an eye co-ordination problem. If the child loses convergence, and reading becomes too tiring, this can lead to double vision.

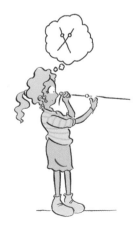

Testing for focusing and convergence

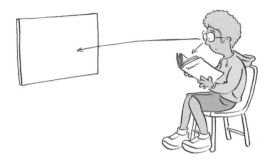

This test is quite simple. Ask the child to read some text – first, looking downward using the normal reading distance, and second, deciphering some other wording (in a size similar to the average classroom board) straight ahead, as far away from their seat as the board would be placed in the classroom. Repeat this five or six times to see if the focusing deteriorates. If so, then you need to do the shift chart exercise.

Shift chart exercise

There is a simple exercise, designed by Gary Heart, M.D., to train the child's ability to shift their focus back and forth from book to board. The exercise requires two charts which you can download from http://www.vision-training.com/en/Download/Children/index.html. The charts consist of a block of letters in random order. They come in three sizes: two of them will fit on a piece of paper that the child can hold in their hand and the third, a larger chart, is placed on a wall.

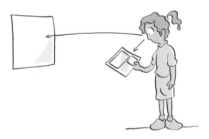

The purpose of the exercise is to train the child to shift their focus between near and far by finding the accurate position of certain letters on each chart. It develops accurate saccadic fixation and spatial location by shifting from the hand-held charts to the wall-mounted chart. This exercise also improves accommodative infacility.

```
O F N P V D T C H E
Y B A K O E Z L R X
E T H W F M B K A P
B X F R T O S M V C
R A D V S X P E T O
M P O E A N C B K F
C R G D B K E P M A
F X P S M A R D L G
T M U A X S O G P B
H O S N C T K U Z L
```

```
O F N P V D T C H E
Y B A K O E Z L R X
E T H W F M B K A P
B X F R T O S M V C
R A D V S X P E T O
M P O E A N C B K F
C R G D B K E P M A
F X P S M A R D L G
T M U A X S O G P B
H O S N C T K U Z L
```

```
O F N P V D T C H E
Y B A K O E Z L R X
E T H W F M B K A P
B X F R T O S M V C
R A D V S X P E T O
M P O E A N C B K F
C R G D B K E P M A
F X P S M A R D L G
T M U A X S O G P B
H O S N C T K U Z L
```

The shift chart excercise. This can be downloaded from http://
www.vision-training.com/en/Download/Children/index.html

Instruct the child as follows:

1. Place yourself just far enough away from the chart so that it is a bit of a challenge to see it clearly.

2. Look at the smaller eye-chart in your left hand and read three letters in your mind. Then blink as you shift and read the next three letters from the bigger chart in your right hand, also reading them in your mind. Blink and shift to look at the larger chart on the wall and say the next three letters out loud.

3. You have the option to alter the way you read the letters. For example, you can start from left to right as in normal reading. As an alternative, you can read the letters going up and down in columns. Or you can start from the end and work back to the beginning. Or you can select three letters at random and find the next three letters on either the wall chart or the hand-held chart. The ultimate challenge would be to spell names, by reading each letter alternately from the wall chart and the hand-held charts. The important thing is to keep your mind interested and have fun with the exercise.

4. To enhance the focusing powers of your eyes, move both toward and away from the wall chart while attempting to see the letters clearly at the maximum distance possible. Do the same thing with the charts you are holding in your hands. To improve near-sight move the charts further away; for far-sight move the charts closer and closer toward you.

5. Do this exercise for a few minutes, then rest your eyes by palming (see Chapter 15). The aim is to accomplish the shifting process as quickly and as accurately as possible. Exercise for a maximum of five minutes each time. Keep in mind, however, that it is beneficial to do this exercise frequently.

6. You can also combine this exercise with tromboning (moving the image closer and further away while attempting to keep it sharp).

The same action described in this exercise can also be done in other environments at home or at school. Switching from one focus to another, combined with a slight challenge in terms of moving the blur zone further away, is a very useful exercise, particularly when the child is in the mid-range of myopia.

10. Common Childhood Vision Problems

Statistically, about 97% of 5-year-olds around the world have perfect eyesight (Hirsch, 1952). So, nearly all of us start out with good eyesight. However, the environment children frequently find themselves in alters their visual acuity quite dramatically. The prime causes of this are schoolwork and video games.

Myopia, or near-sight, is the most common vision problem. It usually starts out mildly at 1 or 2 diopters. Often it is simply accommodative excess or tired eyes which causes a blurriness of vision when you look up from your book. You may know of people who were prescribed glasses in childhood but never wore them. As adults they have perfect eyesight. This could have been for no more complex reason than that their eyes had a chance to recover without being interfered with.

Myopia is present in about 3% of 6-year-old children when they first attend school. By the age of 15, about 17% of them will be near-sighted. In Asia, this is around 85% by the age of 17, mostly because of the intensive amount of close schoolwork that children are obliged to do. (For a more detailed description and exercises please see Chapter 12.)

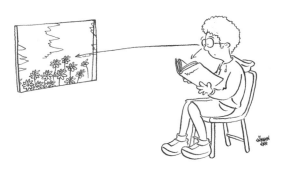

Hyperopia, or far-sight, affects about 6–8% of children, fewer in Asia than in Europe, Australia and North America. Far-sighted children have a resting point that is further away than with other children. Therefore, it takes a lot of visual strength to look at something close-up, such as when reading. There is a misconception that being far-sighted leads to strabismus or amblyopia. In some cases, far-sighted children with strabismus are prescribed very strong plus lenses in order to force the eye to look straight through the center of the lens. These lenses are not prescribed because the child needs them to see; their purpose is to correct the direction of the diverging eye. (For a more detailed description and exercises please see Chapter 14.)

Eye co-ordination is one of the vision skills that is rarely tested by doctors or optometrists. It concerns how accurately the eyes converge on the object being observed. Convergence insufficiency is when the eye converges in front of what we are looking at. For example, when reading, convergence insufficiency will cause the words to seem slightly double, so it requires a lot of concentration. When the affected child gets tired, the words also begin to move around. Fortunately, it is easy for parents to detect this problem and help to correct it. (For a more detailed description and exercises please see Chapter 18.)

Amblyopia, or lazy eye, affects about 2–4% of children. This condition occurs when there is a discrepancy in the vision between the left and right eye. The brain tends to suppress any visual image that is blurry or that turns away, as in strabismus. Amblyopia may develop in early childhood, but may go unnoticed until the eyes are tested. (For a more detailed description and exercises please see Chapter 20.)

Strabismus, or divergent eye, is a condition that affects about 6–8% of children. The cause of strabismus is still unknown. The most common type is esotropia, which is when the eye turns in toward the nose. Exotropia, when the eye turns out, is less common. The eye can also turn up or down and even turn outward at the same time. Strabismus generally responds very well to Vision Training. The problem here is not with the eye muscles; the real issue is the movement of the brain and how it controls the motion of the eye. For this reason, surgery should be considered only as the very last option, since Vision Training is much more effective and gives lasting results. (For more a more detailed description and exercises please see Chapter 19.)

Other visual efficiency and processing difficulties described in this book are also quite common but less well known because they are generally not detected by the common vision test. It is my wish that this book will be a step in the direction of raising awareness about the understanding and treatment of these less well-known vision problems.

11. Are Glasses Really the Best Option?

Most people do not question the widely held assumption that donning a pair of glasses is the best thing they can do for their eyesight problems. Very few parents know what really happens when they put glasses on their children, and why this may not be the best solution.

The optics of glasses

Vision is not static: our eyesight is in a constant state of change. This is a fact that most people are familiar with – for instance, all of us have felt our eyes becoming tired after hours of reading or after a long day in front of a computer.

Glasses are fitted in order to correct refractive error. In other words, the lens is used to focus the image that we see precisely onto the retina. However, glasses compensate for the refractive error in an inflexible way. When you wear glasses, the level of refractive error is maintained constantly for near vision and distance vision whether you need it or not.

This problem is further aggravated, as is often the case, if the prescription is for 100% correction at the exact time of measurement. This means that the eyes need to constantly adapt to the conditions at the moment when they were tested. So, if you happen to have your child's eyes tested in the afternoon after school, their eyes will always be forced to adapt to those conditions. You may have experienced this yourself when putting on new glasses for the first time, only to find that the prescription hurts your eyes. When you complain about this to the ophthalmologist the answer is usually, "You will get used to them in a few days."

What happens to your child's eyesight with this continuing situation? Obviously, their eyes have to adapt themselves by continually replicating the refractive error the way it was that afternoon when their eyes were measured. In other words, their eyesight is forced to deteriorate, just so the glasses will fit.

Why using minus lenses for reading is bad for the eyes

Using minus lenses for reading actually makes vision worse. The scientific explanation for this is that the eyes have to over-accommodate or adjust by -3 diopters in order to read at a normal reading distance. So, if your child wears -3 diopter lenses to correct their eyesight at a distance, but they keep their glasses on for reading, then their eyes have to adjust not only for the -3 diopters that people with normal eyesight need, but also the -3 diopters in their glasses. Basically, the child's eyes are required to adjust/accommodate by -6 diopters for as long as they wear their glasses for reading.

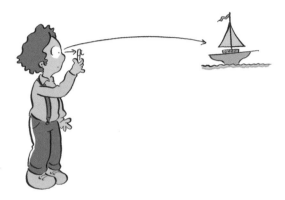

Since the glasses are static, if they provide clear vision starting at 6 meters, then they will be 20 times out of alignment if they are used for reading at 30 cm. If you look at an object 3 meters away, they will be 50% inaccurate. This fact is difficult to get around if you need to wear glasses. At this point in time, it is not possible to make glasses that vary their power as you change from reading to looking out of the window. (Your video camera has the capability to do this by moving the lens elements back and forth to keep the filming in focus.)

This is the reason why using glasses designed for correcting distance vision while reading is bad for the eyes. This additional strain on your child's eyes can only have a detrimental effect on their vision. Instead, encourage them either to take their glasses off or to read while looking over the top of the frame.

The importance of the optic center

The lenses in glasses have only one point of best vision – through the optic center. This means that they are constructed as if you are always looking through the dead center of the lenses, with this point located directly in front of your eyes as you look straight in front of you. When you look through your glasses and turn your eyes in and away from this center point, the lenses become more like prisms. (You have probably seen this effect on photographs taken through wide-angle lenses: the edges of the image are distorted.) This, along with the fact that glasses also have some sort of frame, encourages you to keep your eyes locked into the position that gives the best vision. Furthermore, a frequently used practice to control diverging eyes is the fitting of strong plus lenses. This treatment sadly ends up driving the vision further downhill.

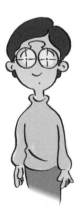

The optic center also plays a role when you use minus lenses for reading. Remember, your glasses are prescribed with the intention of correcting your distance vision. When you look at the horizon, your eyes point straight out through the optic center of the glasses. However, when you read you turn your eyes in and down in order for your eyes to converge on the page. Unless you wear special reading glasses, or have them incorporated into your glasses, the optic center of each lens will be further apart than is required. The result is additional strain on the eyes, and the more you read the greater the damage.

If you wear near-sight glasses while working at a computer, they will be wrongly adjusted for both reading (about 35 cm) *and* the computer screen (about 60 cm). This is a contributing factor to the way that computer work detrimentally affects eyesight.

Does wearing glasses affect the size of the eyes?

Shockingly, there is plenty of scientific evidence that lenses fitted on young primates affects the development of their eyes. In research at a New York City College, biologists demonstrated that wearing a minus lens causes the elongation of the eyeball – in other words, it causes near-sight to deteriorate (Zhu et al., 2003). Plus lenses fitted for far-sight causes a shortening of the eyeball thus making the far-sight worse. This research into emmetropization, the natural ability of the eyes to develop clear vision, goes back to the early 1960s. Of course, the idea that glasses make your vision worse is resisted by the optic industry; just as tobacco smoking is not considered harmful by the tobacco companies.

The objective of the Vision Training approach is to completely eliminate the need for glasses by means of exercises. Our goal is natural clear vision – nothing less.

12. Near-Sightedness

Myopia is the most common visual problem for children. It is also the most researched. For more than a hundred years, researchers have attempted to understand what causes myopia. In 1952, Hirsch concluded that less than 3% of 5-year-olds have myopia. Only when children enter school does childhood myopia set in, and every year sees children's eyesight worsen between -0.30 and -0.50 diopters per year (Bücklers, 1953). The progression slows down in the mid-teens, and earlier for girls than for boys. This, of course, has also increased the myopia rate in high school children.

What causes myopia?

What is it that causes a disturbing percentage of children to become near-sighted by the time they leave school? Often parents are told that myopia is due to genetic factors passed on from family members. Young and colleagues (1969) carried out a study of a community of Eskimos in Alaska. They found no evidence that any of the grandparents had suffered vision problems. However, among the 21- to 25-year-olds, the incidence of myopia was an astonishing 88%. What had apparently caused the change was the fact that these children had been to school.

So, at least among Eskimos, vision problems do not appear to be inherited. Other studies of native societies have found that when children enter school they start to become near-sighted. Genetic factors do not change from one generation to another, so the genetic theory must play a lesser role compared to environmental influences, such as extended near focus while studying.

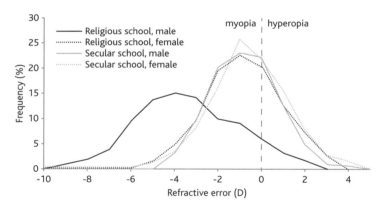

Another interesting example comes from Zylbermann et al.'s (1993) study of Israeli teenagers. Orthodox Jewish boys have to learn the Torah by heart so that they can recite it line by line. As a result, they spend a huge amount of time reading. The boys who attend religious schools demonstrate significantly worse myopia than the girls, who are not required to study the Torah so extensively. This is a good example of how excessive close work causes myopia, since it is obvious that boys and girls from the same family will share the same genetic background. Children from secular schools had milder degrees of myopia, just like the girls in religious schools. We can, therefore, assume this is not down to genes!

Near work and myopia

Extensive near work can increase the risk of myopia, particularly if the work surface is too close to the child's eyes – for example, if the desk or table is too high or the chair too low. I have had cases of children who were too small for the desks provided by the school. I could not get them lower desks, but at least I managed to get them higher chairs. Reading or writing closer than the length of the lower arm, also known as the Harmon distance, may lead to visual stress (accommodative excess or pseudomyopia).

The Kansas Optometry Association (cited in Crane and Crane, 2006) tested 10,000 3-year-old children and found that about 3% of them had measurable visual problems. They tested the same 10,000 children after the third grade and found that, by then, 17% of them were near-sighted. The belief is that this incredible increase in myopia is connected with, among other things, the height of the school desk in relation to the child's physical size. In other words, the children were being forced to overuse their eyes to focus for extended periods too close to their eyes.

This phenomenon occurs particularly during kindergarten and the first few years of school when most children are naturally slightly far-sighted. Progressively, the longer time they are required to do near work causes eyestrain. The typical symptom of accommodative excess is blurry vision when they look up. This is often assumed to be near-sightedness and the child is given glasses. In fact, a study investigating whether glasses were prescribed too readily (Donahue, 2004) found that of 102,508 preschool children screened, 890 children did not have amblyogenic factors (false-positive screenings). Nevertheless, spectacles were prescribed for 174 (19.5%) of these children. Therefore, a significant percentage of preschool children were prescribed glasses unnecessarily. Donahue goes on to estimate the cost of unnecessary glasses in the United States at about US$200,000,000.

Myopic children habitually work at closer distances than children with normal eyesight (Haro et al., 2000), and myopic progression is significantly higher in children with closer near working distances that are less than the normal reading distance (Parssinen and Lyyra, 1993). Some children read as close as 10 cm, at which distance the eyes must adjust to -10 diopters. Others read at 8 cm which requires the eye to adjust -13 diopters. Reading or playing video games at these distances can very quickly lead to accommodative stress. The result is an instantaneous blurring which is not near-sightedness but a symptom of focusing stress (Suchoff and Petito, 1986).

One study found that myopes took significantly fewer fixation breaks than children with normal eyesight at a close distance, suggesting that breaks from reading at close distance may have a protective effect (Harb et al., 2006). This is consistent with findings that even brief periods of myopic defocus (looking away) inhibit the axial eye growth to sustained periods of hyperopic defocus (near work) in animal studies (Zhu et al., 2003).

Many children also play video games for extensive periods at a very close distance. This behavior plays a significant role in myopia. It is even worse if children wear glasses for their games marathons. The reason, as already discussed, is that the eyes have to accommodate not only for the particularly close distance but also for the lens power. Eyes normally adjust -3 diopters in order to read a book, but when you are wearing glasses you have to add the power of the lenses into that equation. So, if the child wears -2 diopter lenses, the change in focus will be -5 diopters. In fact, with a prescription of -2 diopters, the child does not actually need lenses to read, since they can see perfectly clearly out to 50 cm, which is about arm's length for most children.

Can eyesight be trained?

Indeed. More than 20 years ago, I restored my eyesight to normal from -5.50 diopters myopia, so I speak from personal experience. It took me three months to go from the top of the eye-chart to the bottom.

Everyone knows that sports performance can be improved by training, so if arm and leg muscles can be trained, then eye muscles should be trainable as well. The focusing system of the eye is accomplished by the muscles in and around the eye. Therefore, the function – how you use the eye muscles – is trainable.

With children it is actually quite easy to restore natural eyesight within a week or two. Children's myopia is usually less than -2 diopters, so the physical changes in the eyes are minimal. The main criterion is to make sure it's fun. If the exercises are enjoyable, and the child realizes it is something they can do, then it's full force forward.

How to measure your child's eyes

First, you need to determine the near point and far point of absolutely clear vision. Visual acuity is directly related to the furthest point that the child can see clearly. There is a linear relationship between the distance to the far point in centimeters and the power in diopters needed to correct their vision.

You will need a piece of string about 150 cm long, a card with text printed on it and two differently colored marker pens.

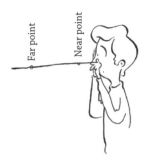

1. Tie a knot at each end of the string so that you have something to hold on to. Hold one of the knots yourself and ask the child to hold the other knot under the middle of one eye on the top of their cheek, so they are looking down the length of the string. The child should cover the other eye with their other hand.

2. Hold the card against the far end of the piece of string, and bring it inward to identify the point where the child starts to be able to see the text clearly. Find the point where it becomes crystal clear. Mark this point on the string with one of the marker pens. This is the child's far point for that eye.

3. Next, bring the card in further to find the closest point at which the child can see the top line of the text with absolute clarity. This is the child's near point of clear vision. Mark this point on the string with the same marker pen.

4. Repeat the whole process with the other eye, using the other colored marker.

5. You now have both the near point and the far point of absolutely clear vision for both of the child's eyes. You can now see if there is a difference between them.

The two near points and the two far points should be exactly the same. If there is a difference, the child has anisometropic vision – that is, one eye has better vision than the other. You need to attend to this condition first. If left alone, they could develop amblyopia in the weaker eye. This means that the brain switches off the input from that eye. Often children are not aware of this, since it develops very slowly.

The near point should be 12 cm or less from the knot which the child was holding. If they have a high degree of myopia, then the near point may be quite close. If this is the case, there is no need to be concerned about it. Usually the near point is not an issue if a child is near-sighted.

Calculate the eye power in diopters

Measure the distance in centimeters from the knot to the far point. If there is a difference, then measure the far point for both eyes. The formula for calculating this is as follows:

100 divided by far point in centimeters = diopters

With this method you can accurately determine the visual acuity of your child's eyes. For example, if the far point in one eye measures 20 cm from the knot, the diopter will be 100 divided by 20, which equals 5 diopters.

Normally a child's near point should be about 12 cm from the knot. If the near point is further out than this, it may be due to far-sight. Whatever the cause, you will need to help the child to perform exercises that will bring the near point back to, or very close to, 12 cm.

String exercise for myopia greater than -2 diopters

If you find that the child can see clearly less than 50 cm from their eyes, then you need to restore their vision back to -2 diopters as a first step. Sometimes there is a difference between the two eyes (anisometropia). If this is the case, you need to do the exercises only with the weaker eye. The first goal is to balance the visual acuity between the eyes.

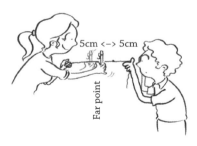

The string exercise is designed to give you a quantifiable method of measuring the parameters of your child's vision. Most people have difficulty understanding the meaning of a diopter reading. The string exercise provides definitive and quantifiable feedback. All you need is a piece of string about 150 cm in length, a colored pen, a bookmark shaped piece of paper or card and a tape measure.

You have already found the child's near and far point of clear vision in both eyes. Now we come to the actual training part of the exercise.

1. Ask the child to hold the string (from the measurement exercise above) under the middle of one eye on the top of their cheek. They should cover the other eye. Move one pen back and forth from about 5 cm before the far point for that eye where they can see it clearly and then out to about 5 cm beyond the far point. Ask them to follow the pen. This will encourage them to focus the eye further and further away.

2. Encourage them to involve their breathing. Tell them to exhale as they move their eyes outward and inhale as they move them back. Get them to do this slowly. You will notice that the child's eyes will start improving in their ability to focus on the pen as it moves further and further away.

3. Test to see what improvement there is after moving the pen back and forth three or four times. Try moving the pen 5 mm further out from the far point. If the child

reports that the text is clear, move another 5mm further away until you get to the last point that is still clear.

4. Make a mark on the string there. This is the improvement the child has made. The child needs only to do this exercise for five minutes at a time, but encourage them to perform it every hour.

The string exercise is exceptionally effective for exercising the focusing ability of the eyes – the medical term is accommodation. You will have constant feedback as the child progresses. In fact, they can improve their vision quite dramatically by doing this exercise. For example, if a child has -4 diopters of eyesight, the far point will be about 25 cm from the end of the string. Move the pen back and forth from 5 cm before the far point to 5 cm beyond the child's far point. Once their ability to see the pen has improved enough to see it 8 cm further away than before, the child will have regained a full 1 diopter of eyesight and their eyes will now have a prescription of only -3 diopters.

The string exercise is the most effective method of retraining the focusing system of the eyes. When the child can see clearly out to 65 cm on the string, it means their visual acuity is -1.50 diopters.

Along the way, you will need to gradually reduce the power of the child's glasses. Alternatively, start out with the child wearing older, less powerful glasses. You know the glasses are too strong when the child can see the second to last line of the eye-chart (20/20 or 6/6). The line does not need to be clear, just readable. The new glasses need to be strong enough for them to be able to read the fourth line from the bottom (20/30 or 6/7.5) – that is, about 10% less powerful. If you want to improve the child's eyesight, it is important to always keep the lens power slightly lower than the actual prescription so the eyes can continue to improve. Remember, their eyes need to adjust to whatever the strength of the lens power in the glasses. You want the eyes to improve by compensating for less lens power; adjusting to stronger lenses will just make their eyesight worse.

Exercise to restore distance vision

When the child has reached arm's length (approximately 65 cm) on the string, then it is easier to use an eye-chart on the wall. You can download eye-charts from www.vision-training. com/en/Download/Download.html. The chart is formed from two A4 pages which you tape together to make a complete eye-chart.

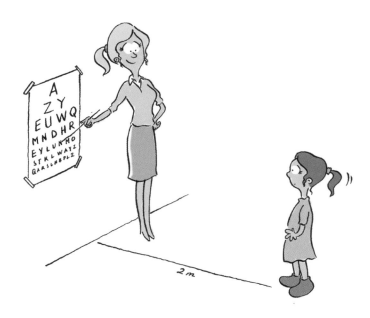

The eye-chart (or Snellen chart) serves as a feedback device for you to monitor your child's progress. The objective is for them to be able to read as many lines down the chart as possible. It is especially effective when the child has just 1 or 2 diopters for correction, because with more than 5 diopters they won't be able to see the first letter of the chart.

1. Place the eye-chart on a wall near a window where there is good daylight and at a level with the child's eyes.

2. With a tape measure, mark out 1, 2 and 3 meter points on the floor and place colorful labels at each point so you can see which distance they are working from.

3. Start the child at the 2 meter point. If they can see the fifth line from the bottom then ask them to step back 25 cm so they can see the letters halfway down the chart. Frequently, the child can actually see the fifth line or better from the 3 meter point.

4. Ask the child to rub his or her hands together for a few seconds and place their palms over closed eyes for about 30 seconds. Palming relaxes the eyes which is helpful in this exercise (for more on this see Chapter 15).

5. Ask them to open their eyes and point to an easy letter (e.g. L, V, N, E) on the upper half of the eye-chart. It is important that the first impression is clear when the child opens their eyes. The brain needs to know that you want clear vision.

6. Ask them to jump from a letter at the beginning of the line to a letter at the end of the line. The jumping makes it easier than looking at the letters in sequence. At this point we want to work down the chart but not read every letter.

7. The letters do not have to be clear – the child just needs to be able to identify them correctly. Jumping around makes it more difficult for them to just memorize the location.

8. Each time you get to the fifth line from the bottom, ask the child to step back 25 cm, until they get to the 3 meter point.

9. From the 3 meter point, ask the child to go all the way down to the bottom of the chart.

10. Do this exercise for two or three minutes only. Make it fun to do and offer lots of encouragement.

Only reinforce the letters that are correct. And expect the child to make mistakes with letters that look the same (e.g. O, D, C and Q are very similar and can be easily confused). If the child does not say the letter correctly right away, then take a break by asking them to palm their eyes again. Small children who do not yet know the names of all the letters can draw them in the air instead.

Sometimes, the child gets stuck on the third or fourth line from the bottom. If this is the case, do not fight the brain. To get around this problem, ask them to move out to 5 or 6 meters from the chart and work with larger letters. When the child steps back to the 3 meter point, the smaller letters will begin to become clearer. This will help to motivate the child to continue.

Eventually, you want the child to be able to see to the bottom line of the eye-chart from 3 meters in good daylight. After that, all you have to do is to check once in a while to see if they can still see the last two lines. If this is the case, then everything is OK. If the child has regressed a line or two, it is time to do the exercise again a few times to get back to them seeing the bottom line.

Many children can read the bottom line from 6 meters. If your child can do this, then they have more flexibility in their

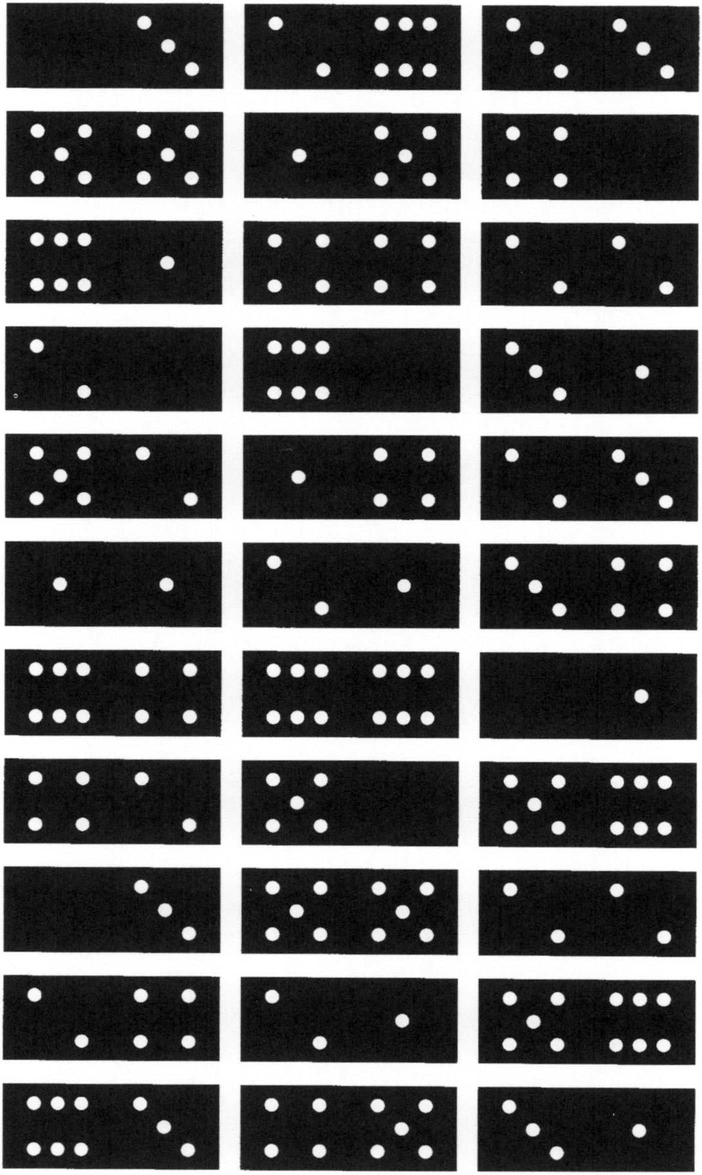

focusing system. This means they have ample resources to draw on when lighting conditions are inadequate.

Domino exercise

This exercise is from Aldous Huxley's *The Art of Seeing* (1942). I have found this to be an excellent motivation booster as well as a way to improve distance vision. Children can very quickly see the domino chart from across the room.

The domino exercise is designed to improve the sharpness of vision and to relax the child's mind and eyes. The objective is for them to get as far away from the chart as possible. Start by asking them to palm their eyes for one minute (see Chapter 15).

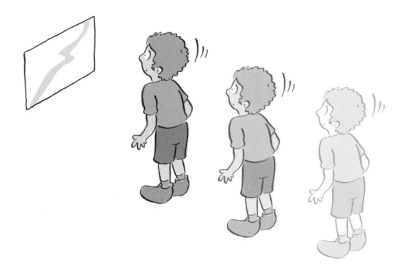

1. Place the domino chart on a wall and find the distance from which the child can see the white dots on the dominoes very clearly. Ask them to step back a tiny bit, so the dots on the tiles are fuzzy but still visible.

2. Ask the child to look at the first row of dominoes and let their eyes run horizontally across them three times. They should notice the white margin, the edges of the dominoes and the dots on each tile.

3. Tell them to close their eyes and, in their imagination, to sweep across the first row of dominoes and exhale very slowly.

4.   Now, ask them to open their eyes and look at one of the dominoes. Invite the child to notice what happens.

5.   When they report that they can see the dominoes clearly, ask them to step back a little so the dominoes become fuzzy again.

6.   The child should alternate between swinging across the chart with their eyes open and closed, all the time noticing what happens. Move the child further away from the domino chart as they improve.

7.   Involve the child's mind by asking them to add up the dots and call out the result as they look at each domino. For example, the second domino has two and six dots, the third one has two times three, so he or she says, "Eight", "Six" and so on.

This is a fun exercise for developing your own distance vision too. Find out if you can see the dominoes from across the room.

Strategies for success

Children are usually willing to do these exercises for a few days, especially if they realize that they are improving. Feedback is therefore of vital importance. In my experience, the best strategy is to find a time when you can do the exercises every hour for two or three days. Remember, the child has to be freely involved. It is not something you can command them to do or do for them. Also, ensure that they know you are looking for clear vision, not just being able to read the letters. There is a huge difference. Just reading the letters does not lead to improvement, but clear vision does.

If the child has less than -2 diopters of myopia you will most likely be able to restore their vision to normal within a few days. If the child has more extensive myopia, then you will need to get them new glasses with lower power lenses.

My advice is then to leave the exercises for a few weeks, and then return to them again intensively for a few days to restore another diopter and then get new glasses. Continue reducing the lens power in steps of 1 diopter until their vision is completely restored.

When the child has regained his or her natural eyesight, then all you have to do is to monitor their visual acuity from time to time. You can do this by keeping the eye-chart up on the wall and asking them to look at it from time to time. If everything is OK, then go on with your day. If not, then schedule some eye-chart exercises to restore their vision back to normal.

13. Can Myopia Be Prevented?

The use of plus lenses for reading and homework

Using plus lenses for reading and homework is an idea that came about by accident in 1904 when a mother visited Dr. Jacob Raphaelson because her son had difficulty in seeing at school. Raphaelson found that the boy's vision was poor, worse than 20/40. The mother promised to pay the doctor when her husband, a printer, was due to return home in about six weeks. For some unknown reason, Dr. Raphaelson provided positive lenses, rather than the conventional negative lenses, and agreed to wait for payment.

The boy used these glasses for the next few weeks. When the father came back, he tested the boy's eyes with different size prints, far and near, and found him to have perfect vision with his naked eyes. He refused to believe that the doctor had effected a cure because the boy's eyes were fine! He refused to pay the doctor and told the mother to return the glasses to Dr. Raphaelson. When the doctor tested the boy's vision, he found it to be excellent. In under six weeks, his near-sighted eyes had been returned to 20/20.

Had Dr. Raphaelson fitted the boy with negative lenses, the boy would immediately have been able to see clearly at a distance. Both the boy and the mother would have been happy, and Dr. Raphaelson would have been paid for the glasses that provided this solution. As the years passed, Raphaelson would have been paid again and again for increasingly stronger negative lenses. This argument, that only an instant solution can be provided and recovery cannot be achieved with a corrective lens, still surfaces in various forms to this day.

Scientists have since discovered what happened to the boy. In 1988, Frank Schaeffel and Howard C. Howland, at Cornell University, set out to find the effect of positive and negative lenses on normal chicks' eyes. They discovered that minus lenses caused the eyes to become more negative or to develop near-sight. Plus lenses caused the focusing mechanism to become more positive or more far-sighted.

From time to time, however, the idea resurfaces of prescribing plus lenses for children when reading. This technique does have an effect with low degree of near-sight (less than -2 diopters). An Italian, David De Angelis, was able to restore his myopia (about -2 diopters) over a period of two years using progressively stronger and stronger reading glasses. His book, *How I Cured My Myopia* (2005), describes the theoretical background and what he did.

However, I do not recommend plus lenses for children. The main reason is that the changes take a long time to manifest themselves, but also lenses of any kind influence the development of the eyes. Schaeffel and Howland's chicken study, as well as later studies with higher primates, prove that beyond any doubt. A New York University study (Wallman and Winawer, 2004) goes as far as questioning the wisdom of fitting near-sighted people with glasses as we know them at all.

Magic Eyes Vision Training works much faster and does not involve any glasses. It is based on the simple idea that you can train the focusing system, just like you would train any muscle for sports performance.

Are Ortho-K lenses the answer?

The appeal of being able to see without glasses is a powerful one. As a result, ophthalmologists have found many ways to approximate this. The most drastic solution is laser surgery where part of the cornea is burned off. Of course, this process is irreversible since you can't put back the tissue that has been removed, plus there are some potentially serious side effects. So optometrists have found an alternative technique which can be reversed.

Ever since contact lenses became available in the 1950s, optometrists theorized that it might be possible to mold the shape of the cornea. Newton Wesley coined the term orthokeratology (OK) for gas permeable contact lenses that reshape the cornea into a flatter shape and therefore alter the focusing ability of the eye. In the early days, this required multiple modifications over a period of months, and the result tended to be unpredictable.

It took decades for manufacturers to develop the technology to create computer-aided rigid gas permeable (RGP) reverse geometry lenses. These were pioneered by Richard Wlodyga. Originally the lenses were prescribed for day wear only. However, from 1993 onwards, special custom made hard lenses were developed to be worn at night.

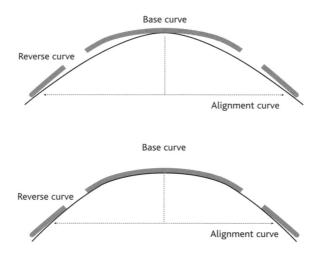

Lens geometry build-up of an orthokeratology lens

Potential problems with Ortho-K lenses

The initial fitting of an OK contact lens has to be done by a specially trained optometrist, because incorrect fitting can cause problems such as centration. Furthermore, bubbles can form underneath the lens when the lens is not fitted properly.

A common problem is that the lenses stick to the cornea and must be released upon waking either by applying eye drops or by squeezing the eyeball so the lens pops out. This procedure often leads to infections because there is a tendency to inadvertently touch the eye. In some cases, corneal ulcers may develop on the cornea. In the relevant literature, reports of infection are not very high. However, infections are, in fact, a common problem, especially if children have to manage the lenses themselves.

Chronic lens binding can also cause severe corneal staining. In addition, exposure to the preservatives found in the contact lens solution is increased since the eyes are closed while the lenses are worn. Because of the problem of lenses sticking to the eye, the Food and Drug Administration (FDA) has only approved a few types of OK lenses for general use in the United States. Also, if a pillow, for example, presses on the eye while the child is sleeping, the lens may exert pressure at the wrong place.

A few years back, the health authorities in Hong Kong called a press conference warning the public about OK lenses. This move was prompted after it emerged that 16 children had suffered permanent eye damage from wearing them.

How effective are Ortho-K lenses?

Research shows that a maximum of -4 diopter change is achievable with OK lenses. So, this procedure is only suitable for mild myopia. Also, it is not a permanent solution: when you stop using them, your vision goes back to what it was before.

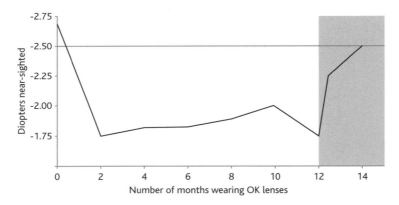

Compared to laser surgery, OK lenses are much safer, since nothing is being cut. It is similar to wearing a corset. While you wear it you look slim; however, when you take it off your shape changes back to what it was before. The misconception among parents is that OK lenses prevent near-sight. This is not the case: myopia comes back very quickly when the child stops wearing the lenses at night.

Compared to natural Vision Training, OK lenses do not seem worth the effort and expense. Vision Training offers a more permanent result and is a lot cheaper. The only drawback with Vision Training is that you have to do the exercises often enough to get significant results. If your child is already wearing OK lenses, they should stop using them a few days before starting the Vision Training exercises. Their eyes will start reverting back after 48 hours, and after a week their eyes will essentially be back to normal.

Your child may experience significant changes in vision when starting Vision Training, especially if their OK lenses were intended to correct more than -2 to -4 diopters. This can sometimes cause a crisis of confidence. One day, the child appears to be making great progress, but the next day it seems like they are back to square one. It is therefore important to be aware of this and focus on the effort the child has made. It is also best to start the Vision Training project at the beginning of a long holiday period, so that the child has plenty of time to adapt. So far, most of the children I have taught who wore OK lenses were very happy to get rid of them and said that Vision Training was much better and lasted longer.

What about drug treatments?

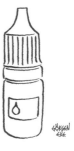

The search for a drug that can prevent myopia has been on for a number of years. Atropine, a nerve agent, has shown some effect in slowing down its progression. Most studies report a reduction in myopia of between 0.25 and 0.40 diopters. Normally, you would expect the myopia to increase by between 0.50 and 1 diopter a year. So, statistically, atropine initiates a significant drop of almost 50%. However, it appears that myopia generally returns when the treatment is stopped.

In a study in Singapore by Tong and colleagues (2009), a group of children were given atropine drops every night for two years. They found that in this group myopia worsened by an average of -0.33 diopters. The myopia of a second group of children fitted with bifocal lenses, as well as being given atropine drops, increased by -0.41 diopters. In the control group, myopia progressed by -1.19 diopters. The researchers reported that "after stopping the atropine treatment visual acuity returned to almost pre-treatment levels."

Atropine treatment also has a considerable number of side effects, including sensitivity to light and difficulty with reading, so many doctors consider it to be unacceptable as a long-term treatment. The treatment is most widespread in Taiwan; less so in Hong Kong and Singapore. In Europe it is considered dangerous, since there are the potential risks of closed angle glaucoma (due to the swelling of the iris muscles) and premature cataracts. There are also potential adverse effects on the retina.

Considering that the positive effects of treatment are minimal and it does not prevent myopia from progressing, it seems that atropine drops are a waste of time and can have potentially serious complications. Also, there is an ethical question mark about putting drugs into the eyes of children who are otherwise healthy.

Back to nature

To prevent myopia, we need to modify the visual environment in which children live. We know that myopia is not genetic. Children who grow up in places where there are a lot of outdoor activities generally have better eyesight. However, in countries in East Asia, where children spend many hours every day doing extensive schoolwork, the incidence of myopia among teenagers is up to 75%. In Sweden, a study found 49.7% of 12- and 13-year-old children were near-sighted (Villarreal et al., 2000).

Try to encourage a balance in your child between near work and outdoor activities. In today's world there are far too many activities that are near and not nearly enough that require children to use their distance vision. Animal studies show that as little as two hours of using clear distance vision can cancel out ten hours of near focus (Napper et al., 1995).

Good lighting is also very important to prevent additional strain on the eyes. Children deserve not only a good education but also a good environment in which to learn. The best kind of light for the eyes is daylight. Inside, lights with 3,500–4,000 K are probably the most comfortable for the majority of people (the color temperature, K (or kelvin), is stated on most packaging). In contrast to conventional energy-saving lamps, LED lights consume very little energy, do not contain mercury and do not flicker.

Ashby and colleagues (2009) carried out a study to investigate the question of whether good light made a difference to chickens wearing lenses. The chickens developed half the myopia outdoors than they did inside with normal laboratory lighting. The researchers concluded that exposing chicks to high illuminance, either sunlight or intense laboratory lights, retards the development of experimental myopia. These results, in conjunction with recent epidemiologic findings, suggest that daily exposure to high light levels, such as daylight, may have a protective effect against the development of school-age myopia in children.

Jane Gwiazda, of the New England College of Optometry, published a review of treatment options for myopia (2009). She notes that several large studies conducted in different parts of the world have shown that the prevalence of myopia in children who experience a greater number of outdoor activity hours is lower than in children who more predominantly pursue indoor activities. So, one of the simplest ways to retard myopia may just be to make sure that your child spends more time outdoors. Time to return to nature.

14. What Is Hyperopia?

Hyperopia, or far-sight, occurs when the axial length of the eye is shorter than the optic components required to focus the light precisely on the retina. This may be due to variations in lens power, increased tightness of the lens or shorter eyeballs.

An Australian study (Mainstone et al., 1998) found that corneal asphericity does not appear to be linked to refractive error in hyperopia. In fact, the study showed a significant correlation between axial length and refractive error (i.e. axial length decreased as the level of hyperopic refractive error increased) as well as to corneal radius of curvature (i.e. corneal radius of curvature decreased as axial length decreased).

About 6–8% of children are far-sighted at age 10. Far-sightedness is less common in China, Hong Kong, Taiwan and Singapore because most children have developed myopia (85% in Taiwan, according to the Ministry of Health).

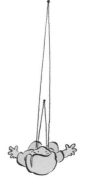

Our eyes have a natural resting point where they will go if there is no visual input, such as at night. This is referred to as the resting point of accommodation. In children with hyperopia, this point of least effort is further away than in other children. This is especially noticeable at school when the child is required to read for extended periods. The extra effort needed to keep the eyes turned inward and to focus close-up uses a lot of energy. Children with hyperopia often get into trouble when they look out the window to relax their eyes.

Hyperopia is usually categorized by the degree of measured refractive error (Augsburger, 1987):

● Low hyperopia is a refractive error of +2 diopters or less.

● Moderate hyperopia ranges from +2.50 to +5 diopters.

● High degree of hyperopia is more than +5 diopters.

How do you know if your child is hyperopic?

When your child is reading, be on the outlook for red tearing eyes, squinting or facial contortions. They may complain that their eyes are tired, they may blink frequently or they may experience constant or intermittent blurred vision. They may have problems seeing up-close and therefore express an aversion to reading. Sometimes eye–hand co-ordination is not smooth and easy.

It is a fact that most babies carried to full term are born mildly hyperopic, with between +2 and +3 diopters. Approximately 6–9% of infants between 6 and 8 months have hyperopia greater than +3.50 diopters. This falls to about 3.6% at 12 months (Menacker and Batshaw, 1977). In more recent but similar research, Meyer et al. (1991) found that 95% of cycloplegic refractions (using eye drops) for children at 4 years of age were +2.83 diopters, suggesting that the upper limit for normal childhood hyperopia at this age is about +3 diopters.

What is important for parents to know is that a child with +3 diopters has a normal amplitude of accommodation or focusing ability, and therefore no visual problem. During the first 10 to 15 years of life, hyperopia decreases through the process known as emmetropization (see Chapter 4). This is a gradual balancing of the visual ability of the child's eyesight to normal.

Types of hyperopia

Latent hyperopia

Latent hyperopia is far-sight which is not manifest but may still require some correction. It is usually compensated for by the normal focusing of the eye. It can be detected by overloading the focusing system by means of a process known as "fogging." This means ascertaining whether there is enough focusing power to see the 20/20 line through a +4 diopter lens. From here the power is gradually increased. Fogging stresses the accommodative (focusing) ability of the eyes to the limit. If the child can see the 20/20 line through a +4 lens, then everything is OK and you can both go home. However, if the child cannot see the chart then they will most likely get fitted with plus lenses.

Latent hyperopia can also be detected under the influence of drugs, typically atropine or other cycloplegic medications. Latent hyperopia is believed to be present in only a small percentage of children. Doctors are primarily concerned with diagnosing and, in most cases, correcting this hidden hyperopia. The main rationale is that plus lenses will relieve the stress the visual system may be under.

Many eye doctors only consider a reading to be true if the focusing system of the eyes is disabled by a cycloplegic. However, I have serious concerns about this kind of measurement. Sports performances achieved under the influence of drugs are not admissible, and motorists are not allowed to drive under the influence of substances that alter visual ability. If you have ever had cycloplegic drops squeezed into your eyes, you will know that you can't drive home afterwards. On occasion, you may actually have to take the rest of the day off and rest. The drops dilate the pupils so you become more sensitive to bright light. It is also difficult to read.

For small children, having cycloplegic drugs put into their eyes is a traumatic experience. And, clearly, if you paralyze the focusing system then you are interfering with the normal function of the eye. Furthermore, cycloplegic drops can have serious side effects and some children are allergic to these drugs.

Manifest hyperopia

Manifest hyperopia, as the name suggests, occurs when the child experiences the symptoms of far-sight and also complains of pain in the eyes. This condition will be obvious when the child is reading, but unfortunately it cannot be compensated for by the child's focusing system. However, usually such children will have excellent distance vision.

Testing for hyperopia

Retinoscopy is the primary method for measuring refractive errors (Rosenberg, 1991). This procedure involves the movement of a light over the eye. When the pupil lights up, the eye has accommodated, or focused, accurately. In the opinion of the American Optometric Association (2008: 14) retinoscopy provides a better understanding of vision and refraction than can be obtained under cycloplegia (Rosenfield and Chin, 1995; Zadnik et al., 1992).

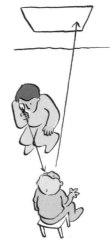

Objective refraction

Objective refraction does not depend on feedback from the child. It is mostly achieved by infrared projection and measuring how the light changes when it enters the eye. The most common methods of objective refraction are retinoscopy and autorefraction.

An autorefractor is a computer-controlled machine designed to measure the physical aspects of the eyes (e.g. dimension, curvature). However, autorefractors are not accurate enough to correctly measure for near-sight or far-sight. Also, because children are able to adjust their vision over a wide range, there is a danger that they simply adapt to the machine. The technique depends on feedback from the child so it is a very subjective test. I have heard from many parents that they've got very different measurements from different clinics – one father told me that his son was given measurements from between -2 and -6 diopters.

Retinoscopy

Retinoscopy provides a much better and more accurate method than autorefraction. This involves using a retinoscope to direct a light into the child's eye and observing the reflection from the retina. By moving a light across the pupil, it is possible to detect the relative movement of the reflection.

Static retinoscopy is performed with the child viewing a distant object with the eyes relaxed. This test provides accurate and replicable measurements of manifest or apparent hyperopia. Dynamic retinoscopy involves testing the focusing response from different angles and distances. In this way, you can get a much better picture of the child's focusing ability.

Subjective refraction (based on verbal feedback) is preferable to cycloplegic techniques (when drugs are dropped into the eye), because it is based on the conscious visual abilities of the child. The eyes respond differently under cycloplegia and the measurement can be less accurate. In some cases, especially with small children, research shows that the cycloplegia test may actually cause the result to be up to 1.75 diopters too strong.

The retinoscope

The retinoscope is an instrument for measuring rays of light as they are reflected by the retina. By observing the size, brightness, speed or direction of a reflection (or reflex) the optometrist can determine if a child has myopia, hyperopia or astigmatism. In 1880, H. Parent (1849–1924) introduced the quantitative refraction test. This made it possible to accurately determine the refractive error using lenses of various powers in front of the eye. Parent coined the term *retinoscopie* (in German, the Greek term, *skiaskopie*, is preferred).

Static retinoscopy involves the child being asked to look at a distant object to relax the eyes. The reflected light from the retinoscope will indicate whether there is any refractive error. If the pupil of the eye illuminates quickly, the child has perfect eyesight for the distance. If the lower half of the pupil is illuminated when a light beam is moved up and down, the child is myopic. With hyperopia, the upper half of the pupil is illuminated. The speed with which the reflex materializes gives a clue to the severity.

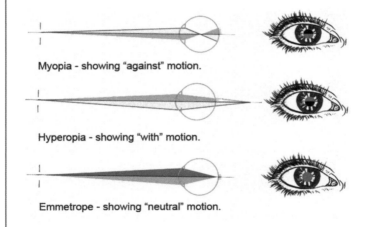

Myopia - showing "against" motion.

Hyperopia - showing "with" motion.

Emmetrope - showing "neutral" motion.

The optometrist will try to neutralize the refractive error with trial lenses until the reflex rapidly fills the whole pupil. The lens power used represents the diopter prescribed.

Dynamic retinoscopy was first introduced by A. J. Cross in 1902. With dynamic retinoscopy, the child looks with both eyes at a small disk attached to the retinoscope. In this way, it is possible to accurately measure refractive errors when reading or doing computer work.

The streak retinoscope was developed by Jack C. Copeland in the 1920s. By making the light beam into a streak, optometrists could now accurately determine the astigmatism meridians. The light beam narrows if there is astigmatism.

Retinoscopy is ideal with children because it does not involve looking into something. The retinoscope test is considered to produce the most accurate measurement. Experienced ophthalmologists often start out with a retinoscope test and end with another retinoscope test to verify their prescriptions.

Plus lenses or not?

Unfortunately, there are no scientifically based guidelines for when to prescribe plus lenses to children who otherwise have normal eyesight but test hyperopic. In a recent study, Cotter (2007) examined the management of childhood hyperopia. She used a survey of optometrists and ophthalmologists to get an idea of the prescription patterns in young children without symptoms. She found that 66% of pediatric optometrists used

+3 diopters of hyperopia as their prescribing threshold for 2-year-olds, whereas pediatric ophthalmologists used +5 as their threshold for prescribing glasses.

There is an apparent lapse or lack of interest in what actually happens to a child when they wear plus lenses. The scientific literature, as well as the recommended practice guide published by the American Optometric Association (2008), stipulates that children under 10 who have low to moderate hyperopia (up to +5 diopters) do not automatically need to be fitted with glasses if they do not have strabismus (one eye turning in or out) or amblyopia (lazy eye).

In fact, there is convincing evidence that putting plus lenses on children is downright dangerous. Studies done mainly by Smith (Smith et al., 1994; Hung et al., 1995; Smith and Hung, 1999) indicate that early optical (glasses) correction interferes with the natural emmetropization process that slowly balances the visual system over the first 10 to 15 years of life. Thus, early prescription of plus lenses may potentially result in maintaining hyperopia throughout life. Many adults report that it actually gets worse. It breaks my heart to see children of 5- or 6-years-old wearing +4, +5 or even in one case +7 diopters.

From a Vision Training perspective, we focus on strengthening the actual focusing power of the child's eyes by exercising the eye muscles that actually do the work. With this approach there are no adaption problems like those experienced with plus lenses.

The fear of strabismus and amblyopia

The main reason that testing is done is due to the fear that children with hyperopia will develop strabismus (where one eye turns in or out) or amblyopia (where the brain switches off one eye).

Prescribing hyperopic children who have strabismus and/or amblyopia with plus lenses dates back to Donders (1864) and Worth (1903). Since amblyopia and strabismus cannot easily be cured by wearing glasses, there is a helplessness that encourages doctors to err on the side of caution and prescribe stronger and stronger lenses, even when there is no apparent strabismus or amblyopia. This belief is, in part, supported by a randomized control trial done by Atkinson et al. (1996) where they had three groups of 7- to 9-month-old children, including one group with hyperopia greater than or equal to +3.50 diopters and a control group with no hyperopia. At 4 years of age, those with initial higher hyperopia in infancy were 13 times more likely to become strabismic and six times more likely to become amblyopic than children with less hyperopia. This appeared to be convincing evidence that hyperopic children with more than +3.50 diopters are at risk of developing strabismus. If you convert the 13 times higher risk into a percentage, it is even more alarming. Consequently, draconian measures are often employed, such as using eye drops until the child can tolerate the strong glasses. One mother told me that her daughter was sick for two days before she could wear her new glasses. It can't be right that children have to get used to glasses that they apparently don't need.

In a later study by Ingram et al. (1990 and 2000), and one done by the Atkinson group (2000), it was found that wearing glasses in infancy and early childhood does not appear to reduce the incidence of esotropia or strabismus.

Of course, if either amblyopia or strabismus is detected, then these conditions should be treated actively – and not just by using eye-patches or half-size glasses. Glasses are passive and do nothing, or at best just compensate for the divergence of the eyes. The eyes still turn when the child removes their glasses.

Vision Training has up to 80% success rate for treating strabismus. Here are a few studies:

- Chryssanthou (1974) reviewed the cases of 27 patients with intermittent exotropia (ages 5 to 33) who received orthoptic treatment. A total of 89% of patients showed definite improvement, with 66.6% graded "excellent" or "good" six months to two-and-half years following termination of orthoptic treatment.

- Etting (1978) reported a 65% overall success rate in patients with constant strabismus (57% of esotropes and 82% of exotropes), an 89% success rate with intermittent strabismus (100% of esotropes and 85% of exotropes) and a 91% success rate when retinal correspondence was normal.

- Wick's (1987) retrospective examination was performed on the records of 54 patients who had undergone treatment for accommodative esotropia. The patients were classified based on the Duane classification of degree of esotropia. Over 90% of the patients achieved total restoration of normal binocular function with treatment.

Plus lenses for hyperopia are primarily prescribed to relieve the visual stress of reading for long periods (sustained accommodation). All the plus lenses do is to move the near point inward by way of magnification. The lenses are passive and do absolutely nothing for the hyperopia. Reading may be more comfortable and the child may be able to read for longer periods of time because the eyes do not need to work so much. However, the risk is that the child's eyes adapt to the glasses, resulting in the prescribing of stronger and stronger lenses. The same phenomena is experienced by people who start to wear reading glasses for presbyopia: they usually experience a worsening of their distance vision as well as needing ever higher lens power for near work.

What should a child be able to see?

The main problem with hyperopia is the stress caused by near work. A child of less than 12 years of age should be able to read 3 point print less than 10 cm from their eyes and all the way out to arm's length. If your child can't read a story book held just 10 cm from their eyes, as well as at arm's length, then you need to do some exercises to help them regain the normal function of their eyes.

While writing this chapter, I had two girls in one of my Vision Training classes. One little 5-year-old came with her mom. The girl was tested to wear +5 but was actually wearing +4 diopters. In cases like this, it is important for the parents to know what the child can actually see without the glasses. It is all too easy to simply put the glasses on, in many cases against the will of the child, without understanding the full implications.

I devised a simple game for her to play without wearing her glasses. We threw a handful of colorful beads on the floor. The little girl had a great time finding the different colors. She also learned that one of the colors was called mint green. The main purpose of the game was to show mom how far and how near she could see a 2 mm mint green bead.

The other girl was 10 years old and had been wearing progressively stronger and stronger plus lenses for about four years. When we tested her visual ability without glasses, her parents were very surprised to learn their daughter could name all the letters on the third to last line of the eye-chart. This line is just 5% less than perfect eyesight and no glasses are needed. The girl could also read very small 3 point print about 8 cm from her nose. So the question is: why was she prescribed glasses? Her parents decided that they would let their daughter go to school without her glasses since it was evident that she would have no problems reading the classroom board. The girl came back two days later with a big smile and shiny bright eyes. Of course, she can always put the glasses back on if they are truly needed.

In a paper titled "Weaning children with accommodative esotropia out of spectacles: a pilot study," Hutcheson and colleagues (2003) concluded that some children with esotropia (one eye turning in) could successfully discontinue wearing their glasses. By gradually reducing the power of the lenses more children could possibly discontinue wearing their glasses earlier. Furthermore children who were not able to discontinue wearing their glasses completely, had a reduction in their under correction angle of esotropia. They were also able to control their esotropia with less powerful plus prescription.

More care is needed when managing the eyesight of children fitted with hyperopic plus lenses. If lenses are really needed, then an effort has to be made to reduce the lens power as the child grows up, as well as applying other effective treatment methods like Vision Training.

Exercises for children with hyperopia

The basic principle in treating the most common types of hyperopia is to develop more flexibility and generate more stamina in the visual system. Everyone knows that practicing your tennis serve or golf swing will improve your performance. If you decided to run a marathon, you would not expect to be able to do so until you first got yourself into shape. If you did train and develop the necessary muscle power and stamina, you could probably run a marathon. You may not win the race, but you could complete it.

The most effective strategy is to develop strength in the eyes so that they can focus near or far as needed. The simplest way to do this is to use them to look at really small things up-close. It is common knowledge that muscles develop if they are trained. It is the basis for all physical training and, of course, it works just as well with the eyes.

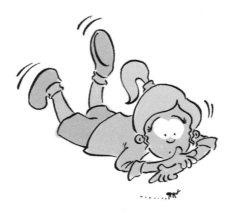

In my Magic Eyes classes for children, I illustrate this point to parents in the following way: "If you are hyperopic or far-sighted, all you need to do is go to the park and lay down flat on your stomach and look the ants in the eye. In other words, look at something really small and really close. If you do this often enough, the chances are that your visual system will build up stamina and flexibility so that reading becomes easy." One father in Taiwan told me that his son could see not only the ants but also their antennae. Now, that's great near vision!

A 9-year-old boy came to one of my Magic Eyes workshops for children in Munich. He said that he did not think he needed to go to an eyesight class because there was nothing wrong with his eyes. I told him that, since he was here anyway, we might as well find out how good his eyes were. He proceeded to read the bottom line of the eye-chart from the appropriate distance. I then asked him to show me how close he could read 3 point print. He could read that from about 8 cm from his eyes. There was obviously no problem with his distance vision or his near vision; however, his mother was very worried because he had been prescribed +3 diopters. Luckily, this boy was independent enough to refuse to wear the glasses and trust his own experience and not be obedient and follow external advice.

Another example involved a 9-year-old girl. After the first three-hour Magic Eyes workshop, she did not wear her glasses during the day but in the evening, before going to bed, she wanted to read a story to her cousin. She found that the print in the book was too small so she needed her reading glasses. Now, that is crazy: imagine a 9-year-old needing reading glasses like her grandmother! Fortunately, there is a very simple exercise to train the eyes to read small print. It was actually developed for people who need reading glasses in their old age but it works equally well with children (see the reading smaller and smaller print exercise on page 135).

What about children who are too young to read?

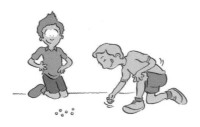

If a young child has no apparent eye co-ordination problem or difference in eyesight between the eyes, then the best thing is to find out what they can actually see, especially close-up and small objects. As described above, you can find this out "accidentally" by dropping a handful of small and colorful beads on the floor. The game is to find them all and, in doing so, the parents should watch the child and observe how far away they can see the beads.

Another game is to play a version of the French park game, boules. For this you will need a collection of colorful balls, and the object is to hit the ball that is furthest away. The child will have to use their ability to see the distant ball well enough to hit it. The parents then get some idea of what the child can see in the distance. Another way is to point out objects in the distance and notice if the child can see the bird in the tree or the airplane in the sky.

If your child has difficulty reading small print

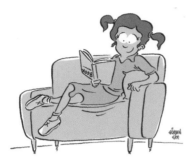

If a child can't read 3 point text, then we need to do something about it. We need to train the focusing system of the eye to identify progressively smaller and smaller text. This is the same exercise that is effective for presbyopia (the need for reading glasses).

Reading smaller and smaller print exercise

First, print out the text below, which progressively drops in point size. The exercise should be done in a place where there is good daylight.

Teacher: Maria please point to America on the map.
Maria: This is it.
Teacher: Well done. Now class, who found America?
Class: Maria did.

A: Did you hear that a baby was fed on elephant's milk and gained 20 pounds in a week?

B: That's impossible. Whose baby?

A: An elephant's.

An elementary school teacher sends this note home to all parents on the first day of school:

"If you promise not to believe everything your child says happens at school, I will promise not to believe everything your child says happens at home."

Teacher: Tell me a sentence that starts with an "I".

Student: "I" is the ...

Teacher: Stop! Never put "is" after an "I". Always put "am" after an "I".

Student: OK. I am the ninth letter of the alphabet.

Two factory workers are talking.

The woman says, "I can make the boss give me the day off."

The man replies, "And how would you do that?"

The woman says, "Just wait and see." She then hangs upside-down from the ceiling.

The boss comes in and says, "What are you doing?"

The woman replies, "I'm a light bulb."

The boss then says, "You've been working so much that you've gone crazy. I think you need to take the day off."

The man starts to follow her and the boss says, "Where are you going?"

The man says, "I'm going home, too. I can't work in the dark."

Two cows are standing in a field.

One says to the other, "Are you worried about Mad Cow Disease?"

The other one says, "No, It doesn't worry me. I'm a horse!"

A: Meet my newborn brother.

What Is Hyperopia?

B: Oh, he is so handsome! What's his name?

A: I don't know. I can't understand a word he says.

Q: What goes Oh, Oh, Oh?

A: Santa Claus walking backwards.

Q: What do elephants have that no other animal has?

A: Baby elephants.

Q: What do you call a hippie's wife?

A: Mississippi.

Q: What did the ocean say to the beach?

A: Nothing, it just waved!

Teacher: Today, we're going to talk about the tenses. Now, if I say "I am beautiful," which tense is it?

Student: Obviously, it is the past tense.

An Englishman went to Spain on a fishing trip. He hired a Spanish guide to help him find the best fishing spots. Since the Englishman was learning Spanish, he asked the guide to speak to him in Spanish and to correct any mistakes in his usage.

They were hiking on a mountain trail when a very large, purple and blue fly crossed their path. The Englishman pointed at the insect with his fishing rod, and said, "Mira el mosca!" The guide, sensing a teaching opportunity, replied, "No, senor, 'la mosca'... es feminina."

The Englishman looked at him, then back at the fly, and then said, "Good heavens, you must have incredibly good eyesight."

Turn the page upside down and instruct the child as follows:

1. Let your eyes sweep across the white space between the printed lines. Continue this zig-zag sweep all the way to the bottom of the page.

2. As you sweep across the lines, imagine that the background is brilliant white – like sunlight reflecting on water or snow.

3. When you get to the bottom of the page, turn it right side up and notice how many paragraphs you can now read with smaller print. The first goal is to be able to read the bottom paragraph.

4. Continue sweeping across the lines for 5 minutes or until you get to the smallest print size.

Bringing the near point of clear vision closer

To find the child's near point of clear vision, ask them to look at this paragraph. Move the text to where they can see it very clearly. This is their near point of clarity. If this is more than 15 cm from their eyes then you need to train them to bring it closer. To bring the near point of clear vision inward, first move the text in a fraction closer, so the words begin to blur. Then move the text back and forth like a trombone player. The child should notice that their eyes begin to focus closer.

Alternatively, you can ask the child to do the exercise by moving the text closer and closer.

Balancing near vision

In many cases there is a difference in the near point from eye to eye. This can lead to headaches. Check the balance of the child's eyes by asking them to look at some text. Place it where they can see it clearly with both eyes. Then ask them to close their left eye and state whether it is still clear. If you need to move the text to keep it clear then the child has a different near point distance between the left and right eyes. Do the same thing with the right eye. To balance the reading distance, ask the child to close the eye that has the closest reading distance. Move the text to a point where the child can see it clearly and begin to move it back and forth (in a trombone movement) until both eyes have the same reading distance.

Alternatively, the reading exercise can be done by moving the text closer and closer.

Developing range

For hyperopic children the most important factor is to develop accommodation amplitude, or range of focusing. When the child can read the smallest paragraph (or the next smallest) from the reading smaller and smaller print exercise above, begin to move the text back and forth, in a trombone movement, until they can read the small print from arm's length all the way in to about 12 cm from their eyes. You want the child to have extra capacity so they will not notice when they get tired and their near point begins to drift out. Finally, the child needs to practice reading small print in different kinds of light.

What if distance vision is lost as well?

By definition, hyperopia means far vision. In other words, children ought to have great distance vision. However, some children actually lose their normal distance vision because their eyes adapt to plus lenses. This disturbing finding results from research by Schaeffel and colleagues (1988). In effect, the lenses become part of what controls the growth of the child's eye. Research shows that wearing plus lenses actually makes the hyperopia worse.

This phenomenon is often a cause of great confusion to parents. Far-sight means that you can see things far away. Often the child has had absolutely no problem before wearing the plus lenses – so what happened? Plus lenses are actually quite damaging to the visual system, especially when the power is more than +2 diopters. Adults wearing plus lenses for presbyopia also notice that their distance vision begins to fail, and the turning point seems to be +2 diopters. So, the higher the diopter power, the more damaging they are.

Most optometrists are unlikely to agree with this hypothesis. However, one optometrist, Merrill Allen (n.d.), has written about this in his article "How to eliminate hyperopia":

> When I'm in the mall, I see thick glasses on small children and I have to control myself. I know that wearing those glasses blocks emmetropization. If Mom would put the glasses on the child only in the afternoon, the child would grow out of his/her hyperopia and require several spectacle power reductions. If the child's correction is less than the refractive error, he/she will grow out of the need for those glasses and soon weaker lenses will be needed.

How to restore distance vision to normal

There is an old and trusted exercise which was used by William Bates, M.D. more than a hundred years ago. First, you need to know you child's visual acuity, or how well they see at a distance. For that you need an eye-chart. You can download one from www.vision-training.com/en/Download/Download. html. Choose any color the child likes and print it out. It is made of two A4 sheets of paper which you tape together to make your eye-chart. These charts are half size and are designed for use from 3 meters. For accurate testing, you need a chart designed for 6 meters. For our purpose, the half-size chart is good enough since we just need some feedback on what the child can see.

Place the eye-chart where there is good daylight and measure out 1 meter, 2 meters and 3 meters, and place one, two or three sticky dots, respectively, on the floor at each point. You are now ready to test your child's distance vision.

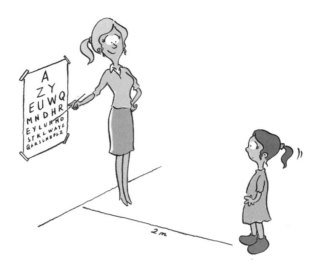

1. Ask the child to stand on the three dots marker. First test the right eye. What is the smallest line they can read? The letters do not have to be clear – they just need to be able to read them. Notice which line they are on and note down the number so you can monitor any improvements.

2. Test the left eye in the same way and write down the smallest line the child can read. It is normal for a child to be able to read the bottom line of the eye-chart from a distance of 3 meters. The second line from the bottom is the 20/20 line (in metric it will be 6/6) – it is considered normal vision. Children with good eyesight can actually see the bottom line on the reduced eye-chart from 6 meters or more. By repeating this exercise, all children can learn to do this.

3. If there is a difference between the left and right eye, then repeat the exercise with just the weaker eye until the child can see the same line with both eyes. When they use both eyes it may be possible to see clearer or smaller letters. This balances the child's visual acuity.

4. Next, ask the child to rub their hands together to warm them up and cover their closed eyes with their palms for about 30 seconds – that is, perform the William Bates palming exercise (see Chapter 15).

5. When they are ready, ask the child to open their eyes and look again at the eye-chart. Start by pointing to large letters on the upper half of the chart, so the first letter you point to should be absolutely clear to the child. This is important, since the brain needs to get the message that the goal is natural clear vision.

6. As the child calls out the letter, point to another letter at the end of the same line. Moving from letter to letter in this way is more difficult for the child than reading out an entire line. Our goal is to motivate the child. Continue jumping from left to right down the chart until the child can't name the letter. Only reinforce the letters that are correct and do not slow down. Show excitement about even small progress.

7. Start with simple letters like H, V, L, N, E and T, as they are easier to see. The aim is to progress down the chart, not to name every letter.

8. Do this exercise with the child for about five minutes, then take a break for an hour or so. Let their eyes rest and restore energy.

9. If there is still a difference between the left and right eye, then repeat the exercise once again with just the weaker eye until the child can see the same line with both eyes.

10. The goal is to see the bottom line in good daylight (not in the sun). When this happens the child's distance vision will be restored.

If the child is excited about this exercise and wants to develop their eagle eyes, then continue until he or she can see the bottom line from a distance of 5 or 6 meters.

Sometimes the child might get stuck on a particular line. Rather than struggle, move to the 5 or even 6 meter point and do the exercise from there with larger letters. When you step back to the 3 meter mark, the child will be surprised that the letters are now clearer and the line below the troublesome line is now visible.

When the child can see the bottom line, then all you have to do is to maintain that ability. Simply test them once in a while. If the child can still see the bottom line from 3 meters then their vision is fine. If they have gone up a line or two, then it is time to do the exercise again to maintain their natural vision. Remember, the environment has an impact on the child's vision. Lots of schoolwork or reading are factors that lead to loss of distance vision, not only wearing plus lenses.

15. How to Relax the Eyes

There are many causes of eyestrain. For example, focusing on a book (or a computer) for long periods of time requires the visual system to lock your eye muscles to the distance from your eyes to the page. In addition, you need to factor in the extra accommodation demand (-3 diopters) needed to look at something close-up.

The default setting of the eyes is to look into the distance. When you are reading or working at a computer for long periods of time, the visual system can become overworked (accommodative excess) and your eyes get stressed, tired and eventually painful.

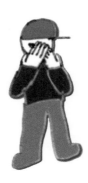

Palming

The simplest way to relax your eyes is to do the palming exercise developed by William Bates, M.D. The theory is that vision problems come about because of mental strain. His remedy is "palming" your closed eyes with your hands.

1. Rub your hands together vigorously for a few seconds.

2. Link the first joint of your little fingers together.

3. Put your hands on as if they were a pair of glasses covering your closed eyes.

4. Relax your shoulders and breathe deeply, exhaling slowly for about 30 seconds at a time.

If you see shadows floating about or sparks of light then your eyes are stressed; solid black indicates perfectly relaxed eyes. When you open your eyes they will feel more relaxed.

Chinese acupressure

In the 1950s, a series of acupressure exercises were introduced to schools in China to prevent myopia. The following exercise is based on the original but with some enhancements. There are ten steps in this exercise. The purpose is to get the energy flowing through your eyes and head. You may notice that some of the points are tender. This indicates that energy is not flowing well at that energy point. The massage movement will start things moving again and you will feel a wonderful freshness and openness.

1. The first point – bladder meridian B2, which improves all eye problems – is located at the top of the nose and up under the eyebrow. Use the tip of your thumb and place it as close as possible

to the inner corner of the eye and press upward. You will sense a tender spot right where the point is located. Rotate in six to eight clockwise circular movements. Alternatively, you can simply press and release several times.

2. The second point – bladder meridian B1, which also improves all eye problems – is located on each side of the top of the nose, right where the bridge of your glasses normally rest. Use your thumb and index finger and grip the root of your nose. Make circular clockwise movements. Alternatively, you can just press and release.

3. The third point – stomach meridian ST 3, which improves cataracts and swelling under the eyes – is located on the cheekbone at the same level as your nostrils, about one and one half fingers outward. Use three fingers and you are sure to touch this point. Make circular clockwise movements. Alternatively, you can just press and release.

4. The fourth step involves several acupuncture points along the bone over your eyes (gallbladder GB 2 and triple warmer). Begin where we found

the first point, then move out in small steps across the bone to the outer corner of the eye making circular clockwise movements.

5. Next comes the bone under the eye. At the inner corner of the eye we have the first point of the bladder meridian. Directly under the center of the eyeball we have the first point of the stomach meridian, ST 1, which relieves red eyes, night-blindness, too many tears and also near-sight. The easiest way to do this is to use four fingers and press down and release on the edge of the bone. Sometimes you will feel a wonderful coolness flowing down over your eyes, indicating the flow of energy.

6. The next step is the gallbladder GL 1 point, located at the outer corners of the eye. Massage with clockwise circular movements.

7. Next move to the hairline to the TW 22 point on the triple warmer. Massage with clockwise circular movements.

8. Move a bit further back, placing your fingers on an imaginary vertical line moving up from the ears. Massage the four points along the gallbladder

meridian with clockwise circular movements.

9. This next move is often referred to as the "tiger climbing the mountain." Open and close your fingers like claws, just as you do when you are washing your hair. Start from the hairline and move up and back toward the center of the head, using one long smooth movement. You can use the soft part of your fingers (if you have long finger nails) or you can use your nails. Put some pressure on to get the energy flowing. With this one move you touch more than 15 acupuncture points on each side of your head.

10. The final point is located at the back of the head just where your neck muscles are attached to the skull. There are some indentations on each side of the head – this is where the 20 gallbladder points are located. Massage with clockwise circular movements.

As you can see, there are many beneficial acupuncture points involved in this simple exercise: you can do for any vision problem and feel the benefits from it, and you can do it as often as you like. It is especially useful to do when you realize that your head is getting a bit woolly as it gets the energy moving around your eyes and head.

Hot and cold towel treatment

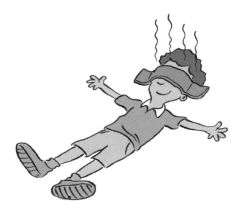

Another way of lifting stress from the eyes is to apply alternately hot and cold towels. For this you need two small hand towels, one for cold water and one for hot water. Dip one of the towels into the hot water (as hot as you can stand it), wring out the water and place the hot towel over your closed eyes for about 30 seconds. The heat will penetrate into the eyes and relax the muscles in and around the eyes. Next, do the same thing with the cold towel, and alternate the hot and cold towels three times. This is a low tech process that will draw out a lot of stress from tired eyes. Do this whenever your child complains about tired eyes.

16. Anisometropia

This is a fancy term for describing when there is a difference in visual acuity between the left and right eye. The image size from one eye is usually larger than the other. Children with good binocular (3D) vision have less than 5% difference in image size between the left and right eye; children with poor binocular vision can have a difference of up to 20%. As a result, the brain will tend to suppress the weaker image. This can develop very slowly and the child may not be aware of it, so don't expect them to announce one morning that one eye does not work anymore.

Children with strabismus are more likely to develop anisometropia, which can lead to amblyopia, or lazy eye, where the vision in one eye is completely suppressed by the brain. The danger zone for suppressions occurs when the difference is more than 2 diopters. In this case, the child may use both eyes for reading but only one eye for looking at the classroom board. Anisometropia may also lead to double vision, tiredness and eventually headaches.

Testing for anisometropia

Visual acuity is usually tested with the right eye first and then the left eye; the difference between the right and left eye is the degree of anisometropia.

It is possible to train the eye with deficiency to equalize visual acuity. For near-sight, do the appropriate exercise found on page 93; for far-sight, do the exercise on page 135.

17. Astigmatism

Astigmatism is very common in adults but less so in children. So what exactly is astigmatism? The most common astigmatism comes about due to uneven tension patterns between the four muscles located at the front of the eye. The cornea is normally a perfect dome. However, if one of the muscles pulls harder than the others then the dome will become distorted and it will be flatter in some angles. This will cause the eye to see several focal planes. In other words, things will appear sharper if you tilt your head in a particular way.

It is not well understood exactly why astigmatism occurs. There are various theories, none of which satisfactorily explain the phenomenon. Some speculate that eyelid pressure has something to do with it. Others cite muscle tension, as mentioned above. Another theory postulates that you are born with it. This is unlikely, however, since the eye grows in size from about 17 millimeters at birth to 24 millimeters by age 14.

There are two main types of astigmatism: with the rule astigmatism is where the axis of the minus meridian is horizontal and the plus meridian is vertical; against the rule astigmatism is where the minus meridian is vertical. The optometrist corrects astigmatism by adding cylinder elements to the prescription.

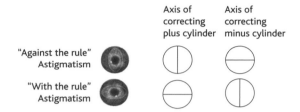

On a standard prescription, astigmatism is described in the second and third columns. The second column indicates the amount of astigmatism in diopters. Less than 0.50 diopters can probably be ignored – it is so minimal that it will be barely noticeable. The third column indicates the axis where the astigmatism is present. All this information is important if you want to manufacture a lens to correct for the astigmatism. Of course, we want to get rid of it altogether.

How do you know if your child has astigmatism?

There is a very simple test to determine whether your child has astigmatism. It is possible to have astigmatism in just one eye, so the astigmatism can be different from eye to eye. There can also be astigmatism at different distances – for example, only close-up and not at a distance, or vice versa. There are even

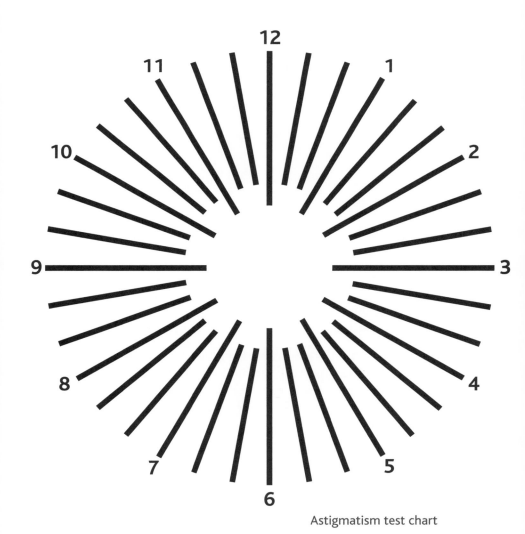

Astigmatism test chart

bands of astigmatism at different distances. It is therefore important to test from close-up to as far as the child can see.

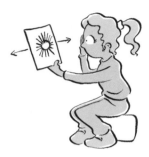

Use the astigmatism test chart on page 155 or download one from www.vision-training.com/en/Download/Download.html.

1.   Ask the child to hold a hand over their left eye.

2.   Slowly move the chart away from them.

3.   Ask them to tell you if any of the lines are different.

Astigmatism can show up as darker lines, thicker lines or shadows, sometimes part of the circle is more gray, and in some cases the lines appear closer or further apart in certain areas. Therefore, if there is any distortion at all, then there is astigmatism at that distance.

Repeat the same procedure on the left eye. Notice where the astigmatism begins or ends and whether it changes as you move the chart away.

Remember, the chart only works as far as the child can see clearly. If you go beyond his or her far point of clear vision, then you are looking at the near-sight.

Having established if there is astigmatism, and where it manifests itself, it is now time to get rid of it.

The astigmatism clown

The clown exercise is exceptionally effective for astigmatism in children. Usually you can see beneficial changes after repeating the exercise just a few times. It is designed to release tension held in the eye muscles.

The exercise is done in two stages: first, do one round clockwise, then ask the child to briefly palm their eyes, and then do a second round counter-clockwise. Ask the child to follow these instructions:

1. Place your nose about 3 cm from the clown's nose. The picture will be too close to see clearly. The aim is to move your eye muscles.

2. Follow the broken line from the clown's nose straight up until you can see the circle at the top.

3. Move from one circle to another in a clockwise direction following the outer perimeter.

4. Next, follow the broken line in to look at the clown's nose and then back out.

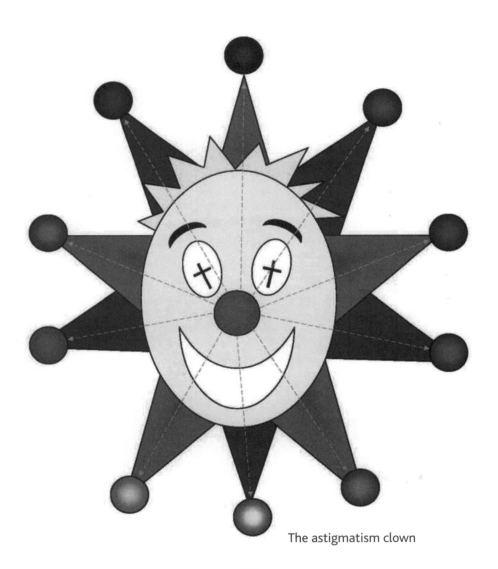

The astigmatism clown

5. Continue moving in and out, stepping from one circle to another, all the way around.

6. Palm your eyes for one minute.

7. Repeat the same exercise going counter-clockwise.

Finally, use the astigmatic test chart and check if there is any difference in the child's vision. Repeat the clown exercise every hour until the astigmatism is gone.

Eventually, you want the child to be able to see the astigmatism chart all the way across the room (when they will have perfect eyesight). It should also be possible to see the chart clearly in angles down to the left and right and up to the left and right. You want to be sure that the child's eye muscles do not produce stress patterns at any angle.

When the astigmatism is gone, all you have to do is to check once in a while to make sure that new tension patterns have not developed. Theoretically, the astigmatism could come back, but it is unlikely. It is like having a stiff shoulder – you move your shoulder, stretching the muscles to release the tension, and it is gone. You do not expect it to come back.

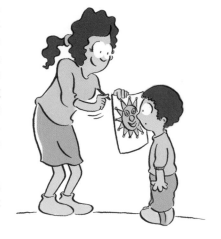

With small children you can use a pen with a light

from behind the graphic. Glue a wine cork onto the nose of the clown so you just have to hold it to the child's nose. Move the light in the direction the child needs to do the exercise, so all they have to do is to follow the light around. This makes it more fun and is simple for mom or dad to do.

The astigmatism train

This is an alternative exercise that works with astigmatism. Begin by positioning the child's nose 3 cm from the square in the middle and ask them to do the following:

1. Start by looking at the train and then traveling around the track as if you were a train. Only move your eyes and keep your head still.

2. Be sure to travel over all the tracks at least once.

3. Making train sounds adds to the fun for small children.

Check with the astigmatism chart afterwards to assess the effect of the exercise.

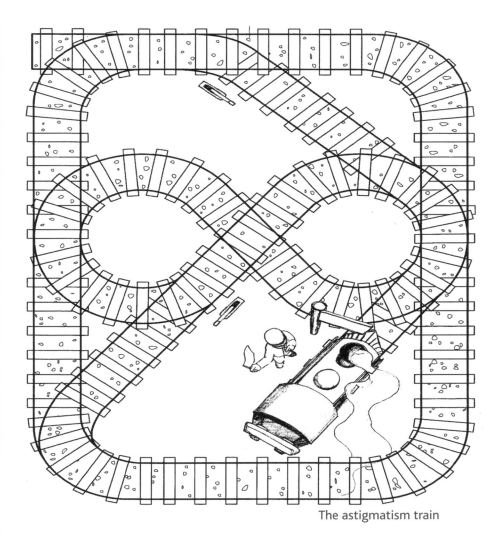

The astigmatism train

What about astigmatism correction in glasses?

The cylinder correction does not make the astigmatism come back if the child continues wearing them after the astigmatism has gone. However, in most cases you can leave the cylinder correction out completely in the child's next pair of glasses – if new glasses are needed at all.

At one summer class in Taipei, Taiwan, one mother came to me and said: "I am so worried about my son's astigmatism when he goes back to school." I told her that her son would not have astigmatism in three weeks' time when he would be going back to school. Ten minutes later she came back and repeated her concern. I told her again that her son most likely would not have any astigmatism in a day or two – and indeed the astigmatism did go away. This story illustrates how astigmatism is sometimes believed to be a condition that is there forever and can't be altered. In fact, it is one of the easiest problems to deal with.

18. Eye Co-ordination

Eye co-ordination is the system that keeps your eyes pointed at what you are looking at. When your eyes turn in it is called convergence, and when they move out it is called divergence. Everyone has noticed how their eyes turn in to point toward an object close-up and then straighten out when they are looking at something in the distance. If there is a misalignment of the eyes, which the brain can compensate for, the medical term is phoria (heterophoria or latent strabismus). A small degree of phoria is easy to compensate for most of the time, but a large phoria can cause eyestrain and headaches and, in some cases, double vision. Reading can become tiring and the child will then lose concentration.

When one eye turns inward or outward, upward or downward, the medical term is strabismus. If the images seen by each eye are markedly different, then the brain will suppress the input from the diverging eye.

Think of focusing (accommodation) as finding the distance at which the object is clear (i.e. defining the plane of focus), while eye co-ordination (vergence) defines the point of focus within space. A triangulation takes place so that your brain knows exactly where in space an object is.

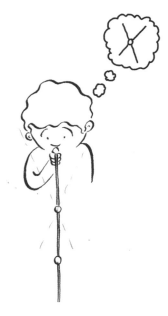

Our eyes are designed to look out into the world. This is their default setting and it requires the least exertion on our part. While looking at a distant object, the lines of vision of our eyes are almost parallel. The closer you want to focus and point your eyes, the more effort is needed to do so. For example, reading requires you to adjust -3 diopters in order to focus on the page you are reading. Doing this for a long time leads to eyestrain or accommodative excess. You experience this as tired eyes, and you may have difficulty focusing when looking up from your book.

The ability to switch from looking at a near object to a far object develops during the first three to four months of life. At about 6 months, a baby may also have developed depth perception, so they will see the world in 3D.

Having poor eye co-ordination makes it difficult to judge depth, relationships and other spatial awarenesses. It becomes hard to concentrate your eyes on the object of your attention, and it is very tiring. You may have difficulty hitting or catching balls, so sports that involve these activities will be difficult or impossible.

Poor eye co-ordination sometimes occurs only at certain angles or at certain distances, so it is important to check this out if your child can't do the eye co-ordination test easily. Various angles should be tested as well as distances beyond 10 meters.

Behaviors which indicate possible eye co-ordination problems include:

- Losing place when reading, writing or copying.
- Skipping lines when reading.
- Using a finger to follow when reading.
- Moving the head when reading.
- Math skills are better than reading skills.
- Complaining of words moving on the page.

Testing the near point of convergence

Near point of convergence testing should be a routine ophthalmological test, but unfortunately it is often omitted. It's actually very easy to do. The purpose of the test is to evaluate how close the child can converge his or her eyes – that is, the near point of convergence. This point should be 8–10 cm from the eyes. If the near point of convergence is further away, the child may have convergence insufficiency, which is associated with attention-deficit disorder (ADD) and dyslexia.

Testing convergence reserves

This measure determines how much convergence power the child has in reserve. Think of this as the additional fusional power the child has to prevent double vision.

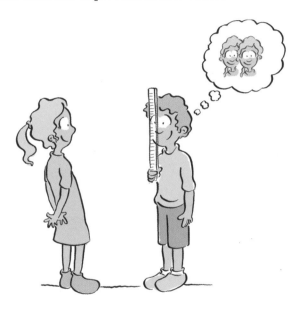

Usually this is measured using a prism bar, which is held horizontally in front of one eye at a time. The child is asked to look at, say, a toy at 40 cm. The prism power is gradually increased until the child reports blurring or doubling of the image. The last prism power reading where the image is clear represents the convergence reserve. This test can also be done vertically. Some children have almost no convergence reserve. This may lead to a doubling of images when they get tired. Doubling may also manifest itself at various distances and angles.

Cover-uncover test

This very simple test can uncover hidden misalignment of the eyes, because heterophoria becomes evident when fusion is interrupted. It is also a test you can do with your own child at home.

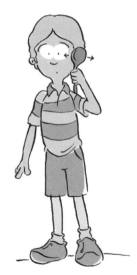

Ask the child to look at something in the distance. Cover one eye with your hand and switch rapidly from covering one eye to the other. Watch the child's eyes. If either of the eyes move, even though they are continuing to focus on the distant object, then there is a misalignment of the eyes.

In some cases, the child is able to control the direction of their eyes while focusing on an object. However, when they are thinking, or in a relaxed state, one of the eyes turns instinctively inward. You can also occasionally see this when the eyes shift from one direction to another, or from near to far. (For more on strabismus see Chapter 19.)

Testing eye co-ordination

Eye co-ordination is very easy to test and to correct if you find problems. All you need is a piece of string about 150 cm long and a paper clip (or a bead).

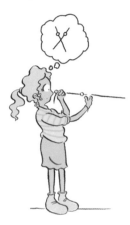

1. Ask the child to place one end of the string on the tip of their nose.

2. Position the paper clip somewhere on the string where the child can see it.

3. Ask, "How many strings do you see?" (There should be two strings.)

4. Ask them to point out where the strings cross each other. (There should be a phantom "X," "Y" or "V.")

5. The cross point should be exactly where the paper clip is.

If the child sees the crossing point in front of the paper clip, then the brain is seeing objects closer than they really are. If the crossing point is beyond the paper clip, then the brain believes objects are further away than they really are. In either case, the child has some degree of eye co-ordination problem. When they become tired, this will most likely increase in severity and may interfere with their schoolwork.

How to correct eye co-ordination problems

To correct eye co-ordination issues, ask the child to move the paper clip to where they see the crossing point. Then move the paper clip back and forth, keeping the crossing point exactly framed through the paper clip. Do this from close-up, as close as the child can see the paper clip, and all the way out to arm's length.

If co-ordination problems persist, use a longer string (about 250 cm in length) and tie knots every 10 cm from end to end. Jump from knot to knot along the string, back and forth from close-up and all the way down to the end of the string. Do this at different angles, so the eye co-ordination becomes perfect – up and down, left and right. In the end, it should be easy for the child and the cross should appear almost instantly.

Finally, to check if there are problems further away, do a street check. Ask the child to stand on the curb and to follow the curb line from close-up all the way down the street. The exact point where the curb line appears to double, or suddenly jump, is where their eye co-ordination is lost. To train distance co-ordination, simply get them to go back to where they saw only the one curb line. Ask them to slowly move their eyes up and down, trying to keep only one curb line all the way to the end of the street. Usually this works quite quickly and the child can enjoy perfect eye co-ordination from then on.

An 11-year-old boy in one of my Magic Eyes classes in Hong Kong said that he was a poor basketball player because he could not get the ball into the basket. When testing his eye co-ordination we discovered the reason why: his eye co-ordination was a mess.

I asked him to get his dad to help him cut five pieces of string, each one about 4 meters long. I told them to tie knots at every 10 cm and mark them with bright colors, to make them easy to see. Then I told him to ask his dad to help him fasten one string in each of the two upper corners of his bedroom and one string in each of the two lower corners (as seen in front of him when he was sitting on the bed). The fifth string was to be tied to the doorknob. Next, I asked him to sit on the bed and to gather the ends of the five strings and to hold them on his nose. The final task was for him to start putting an "X" on all the colored knots. The next time I saw him he was beaming because in his last basketball game he had scored three times. Now his eyes knew where the basket was it was easy for him to throw the ball into the hoop.

Eye co-ordination can also affect reading. Lars' father told me that his son did not like to read; he preferred sports. After fixing his eye co-ordination problem, Lars all of a sudden wanted to read his sister's Harry Potter book, because now he could read for pleasure and without strain. It was that simple. It took an hour and Lars was fine from then on.

Demands in the classroom require a broad range of focusing distances (it is called accommodative amplitude) from book to classroom board and back again, so it is important to check the child's ability to make rapid changes of focus. Both eyes must have the power to focus, as well as converge, at both near and far quickly and accurately.

Some children have difficulty copying from the classroom board to their workbook because they do not know where they are. They have to read from the beginning every time they look up at the board. Normally, you can read halfway down a page, look up and answer a question and, when you look back down again, your eyes will automatically point to the next word on the line where you left off. To do this requires a normal accommodative vergence function. The shift chart exercise in Chapter 9 will help to train the child's ability to rapidly focus near and far, as well as staying on the correct line.

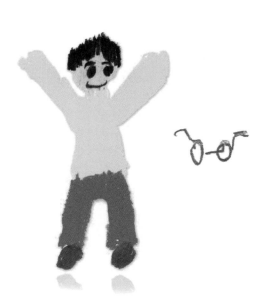

19. Strabismus

Strabismus is a condition where one eye turns in a different direction to the other, which can impair binocular vision. The most common divergence, accounting for almost 50% of all cases, is toward the center, which is called esotropia (from the Greek *eso*, meaning inward). In this case, the inner rectus muscle is too tense causing the eye to be turned too far inward. When the eye turns out it is known as exotropia (from the Greek *exo*, meaning outward). The divergence may be only slight and almost imperceptible to very severe, in which case the pupil is almost hidden in the corner of the eye. The divergence may also occur upward, which is called hyperphoria (from the Greek *hyper*, meaning above) or it can be downward, known as hypophoria (from the Greek *hypo*, meaning down). Strabismus is usually present at a very early age but it can also develop in adults.

If the divergence leads to stressful double vision, the brain switches off the image from the divergent eye, thereby creating amblyopia (or lazy eye). This is the reason why strabismus and amblyopia are often associated.

As described in Chapter 18 on eye co-ordination, there is also a type of strabismus known as heterophoria, or latent strabismus, which is a deviation that is normally held in check by normal convergence. In some people you might notice a slight divergence, especially when they are engaged in internal processing. However, when they focus on you, or some object of interest, the eyes are perfectly co-ordinated.

The medical approach to strabismus is usually to recommend surgery – that is, to cut one or more of the eye muscles and reattach them in such a way that the eye looks straight. The procedure is mostly done for cosmetic reasons. It is quite difficult to surgically modify the way the brain controls eye movements.

If hyperopia is present, optometrists will usually try to control strabismus with the use of strong plus lenses. A strong plus lens forces the eye to look straight through the center and thus makes the eye appear straight. The procedure usually involves the optometrist placing stronger and stronger plus lenses in front of the eyes over time. The glasses do not help the child to see, however, they are merely utilized to make the eyes appear straight.

Another approach involves the placement of prisms in front of the eye in order to correct the angle of sight. Glass prisms become too heavy quite quickly, so plastic prisms are sometimes used instead. However, Fresnel lenses made of plastic are very visible and, understandably, many children do not want to wear them.

Sometimes half lenses, with a line through the center, are used for this condition. This encourages the eye to look straight ahead. Of course, these glasses do very little for the strabismus. When you take the glasses off, the eye still turns away.

In order to truly correct strabismus you need to involve the brain because the tone of the eye muscles turning the eyes is controlled by the brain. Vision Training teaches the brain to do just that.

Testing for strabismus

The ability to adjust for looking from a near object to a far object develops during the first three to four months of life. During that time, an infant's eyes may show strabismus from time to time. This lessens as the baby develops more control over their eye movements.

There are three simple tests you can get the child to perform in order to determine the degree and type of strabismus: the Hirschberg test, the cover test and the cross-over test.

The Hirschberg test

The Hirschberg test involves using a small pen light held at eye level from a distance. Shine the light into the child's eyes so you can see the light spot on the cornea. In normal eyes the spot will be right in the center of the black pupil. The more the eye diverges, the further from the center the spot will appear, and the higher the degree of strabismus. Every millimeter the eye deviates is equal to 7 degrees, or 15 prism diopters. As

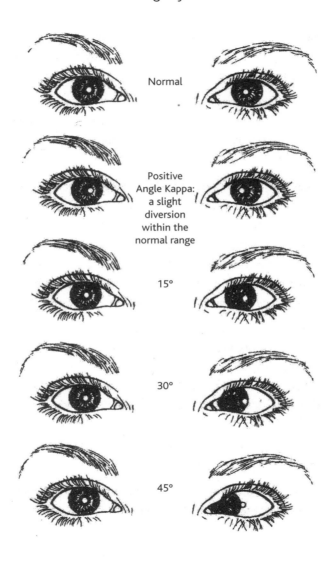

Normal

Positive
Angle Kappa:
a slight
diversion
within the
normal range

15°

30°

45°

explained previously, if the eye turns inward it is esotropia, if the eye turns outward it is exotropia, if it turns upward it is hypertropia and if it turns downward it is hypotropia. Note that a 1 mm displacement is considered normal.

The cover test

The cover test is used to detect if there are any movements in the uncovered eye when an occluder (something that covers the eye) is placed over the eye. Test one eye at a time.

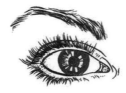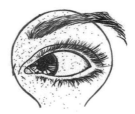

1. To check the right eye, ask the child to look at you.

2. Cover the left eye momentarily – a few seconds is enough.

3. Observe the right eye when you remove the occluder. The eye should remain still. Any adjustment of the eye will indicate a phoria.

4. Repeat the test on the left eye.

5. Also do the test with the child looking at an object far away.

The cross-over test

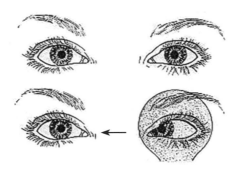

The cross-over test is used to reveal the full extent of the strabismus. The test also uses an occluder which is transferred from eye to eye. The longer the occluder is held before transferring, the more disruptive it is to the fusion. It should be performed for both eyes with the child looking at a near as well as a far object.

1. Briefly place the occluder over the left eye and then move it across to cover the right eye.

2. Observe the left eye as you move the occluder away.

3. If there is latent or hidden strabismus that will be apparent because the eye will turn in or out. When fusion is disrupted, the eye will show the latent strabismus position of the eye.

4. Repeat the test with the right eye.

This test can also be done with a semi-transparent material to reveal if there is latent (hidden) strabismus. If latent strabismus is present, then the affected eye will turn behind the occluder.

What is a prism diopter?

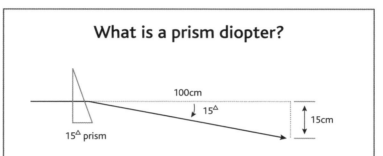

A prism is a triangular piece of glass or plastic. The tip is called the apex and the wide end is called the base. When you look through a prism it makes the line of sight bend in the direction of the base (the angle of deviation).

One prism diopter shifts an image 1 cm at 100 cm. The position of the prism base is indicated by "base in" or "base out" in relation to the nose. In the case of hyperphoria it will be "base out" – the line of sight of the eye that is turned up is modified by the base of the prism thereby causing the eye to look straight. If the eye turns out (exophoria) a "base-in" prism would be used.

Training away strabismus

Step 1

The initial step, and the most difficult one, is to get the brain to allow input from both eyes at the same time. Children sometimes develop a switching strategy so they can swap from left to right eye very quickly. In this case, we need to trick the brain into using the input from both eyes. To do this we use a piece of string.

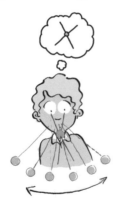

Cut a piece of string about 150 cm long and place a paper clip (or bead) on the string about 25 cm from the end. Ask the child to hold the end on their nose and look at the paper clip. You hold the other end of the string.

Slowly move the string from side to side and up and down. When the child sees two strings, the eyes are converging and there is no strabismus. It is impossible for the child to see two strings and not be using both eyes at the same time. Getting the image of the two strings to appear is an important first step. Ask the child to report at which angle the two strings seem to suddenly appear.

This first step is the most important. Sometimes the child may have difficulty seeing the second string. In such cases I have been successful in using a prism bar (a stack of prisms with progressively stronger and stronger power). By moving the prism bar slowly upward, the child will, at some point, see a second string. When the prism has bent the line of sight to a point where co-ordination can occur, the first step will have been achieved. It is now a matter of slowly reducing the prism power so that the child's brain can take over. The usual use of a prism bar is to check the co-ordination power (see Chapter 18).

Another way of getting both eyes to switch on is to ask the child to close one eye and slowly open it again, all the while looking at the paper clip. At some point they will see the second string. This may require some experimentation, so make it into a fun activity.

Step 2

Now we want to retrain the brain to co-ordinate both eyes perfectly. Ask the child to point to where the two strings come together on an "X," "Y" or "V." Ask them to move the paper clip to where the crossing point is, and then move it back and forth. It is important that the child does this, because we want the brain to accurately identify where in space the paper clip is. Moving the crossing point back and forth requires the brain to move the eyes correctly. They should continue doing this out to arm's length. This can be quite strenuous, so do this exercise only for a minute before asking the child to take a break.

Step 3

Finally, we want to extend the child's ability to co-ordinate their eyes further out and in all directions – left and right, up and down.

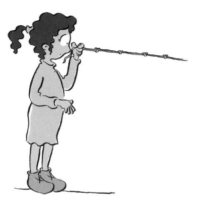

The simplest way to do this is by using a long string (250 cm) with knots at every 10 cm. Ask the child to place one end of the string on their nose and practice the "X," "Y" or "V" exercise on every knot. The crossing point should be exactly on each knot. If not, move the crossing point to the nearest knot using your finger. When the child can place the crossing point precisely on every knot in all directions, it means the strabismus has gone.

Note: These exercises work best with children aged 7 and above. Small children do not always understand what we want them to do.

Dominic's story

"Do I look more handsome with or without glasses?" my son, Dominic, aged 8, asked. "You looked handsome with glasses but you look so smart without them," I said.

Dominic started to miss his glasses soon after he got rid of them, as people used to say he looked good wearing them. He was born far-sighted, so the ophthalmologists said, and was prescribed +7 diopters. He began to wear glasses at the age of 2.

Magically, after joining the Magic Eyes workshop conducted by Leo, he got rid of his far-sight. In three days he was free of his glasses.

On the first day of the workshop, Dominic learned to do the string and knots exercises. Leo stressed that he must do this repeatedly and intensively on the second day if we were to see any quick results. How intensive? Up to 50 times a day, which means you must do it every 15 minutes. Dominic almost hit the target as he did it 48 times.

But it paid off. He was rid of the far-sight problem almost at once. He told me he saw things very clearly without his glasses. We had made it, except for one thing: his two eyes were not co-ordinating very well. The vision in his right eye was better than in the left, so at times the left eyeball would turn in. This worried me as the workshop was over and I felt a little bit helpless.

I managed to speak to Leo over the phone the next day and he asked me to keep practicing the string and knots exercises, as well as the eye-chart, with Dominic until the eyeball would not turn in. Dominic and I were doing the exercises as a team so both of us needed to work hard. But Dominic had to go back to school after the holidays, so we just forgot about the exercises for the moment, as advised by Leo – "Give him a break," he said. "Do it only at weekends." We spent the following weekend practicing the string and knots and the eye-chart. This time we did it about 20 times (I just wanted to make him feel relaxed so I did not push him real hard). Also, I remembered what Leo said: we, the parents, must give the kids lots of praise when doing the exercises. I did. By the end of the day, I almost noticed the change. His left eyeball did not turn in that often. We did the exercises again over the next weekend and I could see that the problem was getting better and better.

After about two weeks life returned to normal. No more string, knots and eye-chart, as Dominic's left eyeball did not turn in at all. It works! The string and knots exercises are very useful. It helps the two eyes to co-ordinate, such that you learn to use both eyes to locate the target (the knots). When you use both eyes to see, the eyeball will not turn in anymore.

I ask Dominic to do the eye-chart once in a while (every two months) just to check his eyesight. He has now achieved the 20/20 (100%) vision. We are working toward 20/16 (120%).

It sounds magical, but it is not. Dominic and I have put much effort into it. You and your kid must work together and be a good team. But, first and foremost, you must have faith in it before magic can turn into reality.

(Teresa Ho, Hong Kong)

My comments

Dominic worked very hard and, as a result, he achieved his outcome quickly. Apart from being far-sighted, Dominic also had strabismus, where one of his eyes turned in toward the nose.

Until very recently, doctors believed that a high degree of far-sight (hyperopia) was a contributing factor to the development of strabismus. It has now become clear that there is no relationship between hyperopia and strabismus.

Dominic was probably prescribed strong plus lenses because of that belief. But just wearing glasses does not do anything for the strabismus. Glasses are passive and corrective only. What Dominic and his mom did with the knotted string was to be active about training his eye co-ordination and, thereby, develop the appropriate automatic subconscious reflexes that produce normal eyesight.

Furthermore, recent studies show that if you put plus lenses on young children you essentially doom them to be far-sighted for life. Fortunately, Dominic still had enough focusing power to overcome the damage that the wear of plus lenses had caused. His mom was quite shocked when she realized that he could only see clearly for less than a meter in front of his eyes. Confusingly, what they needed to do to repair the damage was to carry out the near-sighted exercise.

This is the tragedy of fitting strong plus lenses. When plus lenses become more than +2 diopters, the distance vision is diminished. It does not make sense and confuses parents everywhere; therefore, the need for the near-sight exercise to restore the distance vision. Fortunately this usually comes very quickly.

Dominic is a wonderful example of what active Vision Training can do. He now has Magic Eyes.

While writing this chapter, a young boy came with some of his friends to my Magic Eyes workshop in Ljubljana, Slovenia. Jonathan had first come to the workshop three years ago, when he had one eye that turned in. He and his father trained for three weeks and Jonathan's eye was then straight all the time. This was three years ago, so the progress lasts. About 30% of children may experience a return of the strabismus when they get very tired or get sick; however, the eye will straighten out again when they recover.

20. Amblyopia

Amblyopia is defined as an uncorrectable loss of vision in one or both eyes with no apparent structural abnormality to explain it. It is a diagnosis of exclusion, which means that when a decrease in vision is detected other causes must be ruled out. Once no other cause is found, amblyopia is the diagnosis.

Generally, a difference of two lines or more (on an eye-chart test of visual acuity) between the eyes or a best corrected vision of 20/30 or worse would be defined as amblyopia. For example, if someone has 20/20 vision with the right eye and only 20/40 with the left, and the left eye cannot achieve better vision with corrective lenses, then the left eye is said to be amblyopic.

Lazy eye is a common non-medical term used to describe amblyopia because the eye with poorer vision doesn't seem to be doing its job properly. Amblyopia is the most common cause of impaired vision in young children. According to a German report, the prevalence of amblyopia in children up to age 6 in Central Europe is an estimated 3.5–6%, depending on the threshold definition of amblyopia applied (Institut für Qualität und Wirtschaftlichkeit im Gesundheitswesen Köln, 2008).

Vision is a combination of the clarity of the images of the eyes (visual acuity) and the processing of those images by the brain. If the images produced by the two eyes are different, the brain may not be able to combine the images. Instead of seeing two different images or double vision (diplopia), the brain suppresses the blurrier image. This suppression can lead to amblyopia. During the first few years of life, preferring one eye over the other may lead to poor visual development in the blurrier eye.

Unless strabismus is present, children may or may not show signs of amblyopia. An affected child may hold their head at an angle in an attempt to favor the eye with normal vision. They may have trouble seeing or reaching for objects when approached from the side of the amblyopic eye. Parents should notice whether the child favors one side over the other. If an infant's good eye is covered, it can result in tears.

Possible causes of amblyopia

While it is not known categorically what causes amblyopia, some of the common causes may be:

- Strabismus – a misalignment of the eyes is the most common cause of functional amblyopia. As the two eyes are looking in two different directions at the same time, the brain is sent two different images and this causes confusion. Images from the misaligned or "crossed" eye are turned off to avoid double vision.

- Anisometropia – this is another type of functional amblyopia. In this case, there is a difference in the refractive states (or prescriptions) between the two eyes.

- Cataract – clouding of the lens of one eye will cause the image to be blurrier than in the other eye. As the brain "prefers" the clearer image, the eye with the cataract may become amblyopic.

- Nutritional amblyopia – this a type of organic amblyopia due to nutritional deficiencies or chemical toxicity. Alcohol, tobacco or a B vitamin deficiency may result in toxic amblyopia.

Testing for amblyopia

Children with outwardly normal eyes may have amblyopia, so it is important for all children to have regular vision screenings. There is some controversy regarding the age that children should have their first vision examination. The American Optometry Association recommends that children are tested at 6 months, 3 years, before first grade and every two years thereafter. In some countries tests are conducted every year, in other countries no tests are done at all and in other countries a test is recommended only before starting school, but it is up to the parents to arrange it.

There are objective methods, such as retinoscopy, to measure the refractive status of the eyes. This can help to detect anisometropia. In retinoscopy, a hand-held instrument is used to shine a light in the child's eyes. In this way, a rough prescription can be obtained.

Visual acuity can be determined using a variety of methods. Many different eye-charts are available (e.g. tumbling E, pictures, letters). A child with amblyopia will find single letters easier to recognize than when a whole line is shown. This is called the "crowding effect" and it can help in diagnosing amblyopia. Neutral density filters may also be held over the eye to aid in the diagnosis. Again, it must be emphasized that amblyopia is a diagnosis of exclusion; other possible conditions must be ruled out first.

Treatment for amblyopia

The usual approach for amblyopia is to patch the good eye. This treatment is most effective in the first few weeks (Stewart et al., 2004). The rule of thumb is to patch only for as many weeks as the child is old. If you do not see progress within that period, it is unlikely to have any effect at all. And some children simply refuse to wear the patch. In some cases, the good eye can be damaged because of the patching, so some eye doctors advise parents to cover the amblyopic eye for even shorter periods of time.

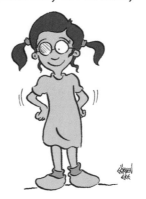

Avoid drastic treatment options like atropine drops in the good eye. Atropine is a nerve agent which paralyzes the function of the muscles in the iris, so that it opens up as wide as the muscle around the lens. It makes the eye much more sensitive to sunlight and, for this reason, it becomes more difficult to focus on near objects. There is also an ethical question mark about putting drugs into the eyes of children who are otherwise healthy.

There are two possible scenarios with amblyopia. The first is that the weaker eye is near-sighted or more near-sighted than the other eye. In this case, we simply do the near-sighted exercises with the eye until both eyes have the same acuity. The second possibility is that the weaker eye is more far-sighted. This is similar to people with presbyopia. In this case, we need to use larger letters in order to find absolute clarity. To do this we use some of the exercises designed for presbyopia.

Wick et al. (1992) reported that with anisometropic amblyopia, a combination of prism, patches and active Vision Training resulted in an average improvement in visual acuity of 92.1%, using the Amblyopia Success Index, formulated by Meyer et al. (1991) as a reference. Patients who had completed the treatment one or more years earlier maintained their improvement. Generally, the research concludes that active Vision Training in combination with prisms, and in some cases patching, is the most successful treatment option.

Exercise for a near-sighted eye

First, perform the string test as described in Chapter 12 on myopia. If the myopia is more than -2 diopters, then perform the string exercise described on page 95 until visual acuity is the same in both eyes.

If the myopia is less than -2 diopters then do the eye-chart exercise on page 98 with the lazy eye. The domino exercise is also useful if done with the lazy eye only (see page 103).

The goal is to balance the visual acuity with exercise and, if necessary, work with both eyes until the eyesight is perfect.

Exercise for a far-sighted eye

A far-sighted eye needs larger letters in order to find a size that is perfectly clear at arm's length. The simplest way to find the appropriate letter size is to use an eye-chart (this can be downloaded from www.vision-training.com/en/ Download/Download.html). The child should hold the chart in their hand, cover their good eye and find the row of letters that is absolutely clear. This does not mean the line they can only just read – it must

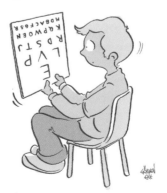

be clear. Note down which line it was so you can chart their progress.

Give the child these instructions:

1. Cover your good eye with your hand.

2. Turn the eye-chart upside down so you can't read the letters.

3. Start with the smallest letters on the line at the top. Let your eye (you are training only the weaker eye here) sweep across the white space in-between the lines. Go all the way down to the bottom of the chart in a zig-zag pattern.

4. When you reach the bottom of the chart, turn it right-side up. Check the line you saw clearly before and notice if the letters are darker on the line below. It is also possible that one or more lines further down are now clear.

Get the child to do this for about two minutes. Then take a break of 15 minutes and start again. We do not want to exhaust the eye; we want to strengthen the eyesight. Continue this exercise until the child can see the smallest letters on the eye-chart absolutely clearly. You have then reduced the far-sightedness to a point where you need to switch to even smaller letters. Always follow up with some praise, such as, "Well done, your eyesight is improving!"

The final aim is to restore the child's ability to read small print. Take a look at the exercise on page 135. The exercise is the same, but it should be done with smaller and smaller font sizes – from 16 point to 3 point. In the beginning perform the exercise near a window in good daylight. This makes it easier and the child will see results quicker. Repeat the upside-down exercise often, just one sweep down. Turn the page around and check the child's progress. When they can read the smallest font size in daylight near a window, get them to start practicing under different light conditions. Eventually you want them to be able to read in all kinds of light, even candlelight.

When the child can read the same size font with both eyes individually and together you are done. Just keep the ability to read small print honed by encouraging them to always look at the smallest print they come across on water bottles and so on. This will help them to keep their eyesight in shape.

Over the years, I have seen many children with amblyopia. In most cases, the difference between the left and right eye has been quite easy to manage with the string exercise on page 95.

Shara's case

A few years ago, I worked with a 7-year-old called Shara in Mexico. She'd had the lens removed from her left eye. The operation was successful, but she had developed severe amblyopia in the eye. The eye looked lifeless and was beginning to divert slightly. Shara had not responded to any of the medical treatments she had been given. In

---

essence, she had given up hope of ever regaining sight in her left eye.

Initially, Shara did not respond to any of the exercises. She had perfect 20/20 vision in the right eye and was consequently using that eye all the time. The other children in the workshop were doing an exercise using eye-charts. In a moment of inspiration, I took down one of the charts and asked her to look at the large "E" about 20 cm from her left eye. She could recognize the "E." I asked her to relax her eyes by palming. Soon she was able to see the 20/200 and even the 20/160 line from 20 cm. This was a tremendous experience for Shara and her mother because it now became apparent that her eye could respond to Vision Training.

The next day, after many short exercises, Shara was able to see even smaller letters with her left eye. Most important, however, was the changing appearance of her eye. It had more life and was beginning to track together with the dominant right eye.

Shara, with the help of her mother, will need to do the exercises for a long time, perhaps years. The good news is that Shara now believes it is possible. After all, cataract removal does not affect the part of the eye that actually sees (i.e. the retina). Vision Training is also effective with implanted lenses.

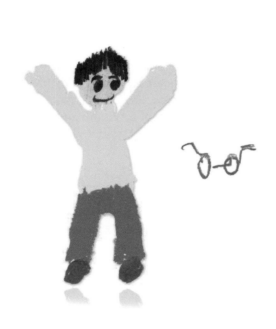

Glossary

Accommodation Changes in the eye that enable you to focus near and far. The lens and other parts of the eye are involved in this process.

Accommodative excess When the eyes focus closer than is necessary. This can occur when a child is overdoing reading or playing too many video games close-up.

Accommodative infacility When focusing speed is slow, the eye is unable to accommodate quickly and accurately when changing from near to far and back again.

Accommodative insufficiency When the amount of focusing ability available is less than normal for the child's age.

Acuity The sharpness of vision, usually at a distance.

Amblyopia Decreased visual acuity in one eye that is not correctable with glasses.

Amplitude of accommodation The child's visual power in diopters. You can work out the amplitude of accommodation based on how close-up a child can see clearly. The norm is age dependent – for example, a 7-year-old should have an amplitude of accommodation of 13.25 diopters and a 12-year-old should have an amplitude of 12.

Anisometropia When there is a difference in visual acuity between the left and right eye. Many children have different diopters in each eye. When the difference gets to more than 2 diopters, there is a danger that the brain will suppress the weaker eye, or one eye gets used for distance and the other for reading.

Astigmatism An irregular shaping of the cornea causing the appearance of shadows or, in some cases, a doubling of the image. Astigmatism can vary from one eye to the other and over distances. When one eye is checked at a time, children with astigmatism can sometimes momentarily overwork their focusing system and still pass a screening.

Atropine treatment The practice of applying drops of atropine into the eyes of children at bedtime to reduce the progression of myopia. When the treatment is stopped the myopia reverts to about the same level it would have been without the treatment. It does not prevent myopia; it just seems to reduce the progression.

Convergence The ability to turn the eyes inward to read. The point of convergence must be exactly on the page. Convergence insufficiency means the convergence point is closer to the eyes than the text, causing it to become doubled. Convergence excess is when the convergence point is further out – for example, behind the book. This also causes a doubling of the image. Both of these make reading very tiring. Affected children often report that words appear to move about.

Diopter A diopter measures the power of a lens. A lens with the strength of 1 diopter has a focal length of 100 cm. The diopter number is calculated using this formula: 1 over far-point of clear vision in cm X 100 = diopter.

Diplopia Diplopia is seeing two images instead of one and is often referred to as double vision. The term is derived from two Greek words: *diplous*, meaning double, and *ops*, meaning eye. Double vision is a common complaint and is often the first manifestation of numerous systemic disorders, especially muscular or neurological problems.

Double vision See **diplopia**.

Dynamic retinoscopy This involves testing vision at different distances for reading or for computer use. A small card is placed on the retinoscope and the child is asked to read the writing on the card. The ophthalmologist can then determine whether the child has perfect focusing or is near-sighted or far-sighted.

Emmetropization Over the first 14 years of life, the eyeball gradually grows to a point where the child has perfect vision. This natural process of eye growth is called emmetropization. An emmetrope is a person who has perfect vision.

Glasses and lenses interfere with this process because the lens impedes the growth of the eye. Eye growth is not controlled by genetics but by what the child sees in their environment. That is why native populations have eyesight that is four to six times better than 20/20. Their eyes are accustomed to the way nature intended them to be used.

Eye co-ordination The ability of the eyes to work together so images are clear, whether you are looking at objects near or far. Co-ordination problems cause double images and make it difficult to read or perform near work.

Eye movement For the eyes to move accurately across the page when reading they must move in unison. If not, the child will see double (**phoria**) and may in some cases switch off one eye in order to avoid double vision. Eye movement skill is often a problem with young readers.

Far-sight See **hyperopia**.

Fixations The instant when the eye naturally stops during the process of reading. There are usually several fixations on any line of text. If the child has too many fixations, reading will become difficult, since letters should ideally be processed one or two at a time.

Focusing See **accommodation**.

Focusing efficiency Being able to maintain clear vision for reading as well as being able to see at a distance.

Hyperopia Most children are born with far-sight (+2 to +3 diopters) which slowly diminishes to become normal vision around the age of 8. Children with far-sight have to use more effort in order to focus on near objects and can develop eyestrain as a result. These children find it easier to read if their textbooks are printed using larger letters.

Lazy eye See **amblyopia**.

LED Light-emitting diodes are a solid state light source used to build TV screens, light fixtures, street lights, traffic lights, etc. LED light is a steady light source that can be produced in all color temperatures. These lights are exceptionally energy efficient and last several years.

Myopia Near-sightedness (also known as short-sightedness) is a common condition that causes distant objects to appear blurred. It can range from mild to severe.

N55 standard The N55 standard is a measurement of the color spectrum of daylight at midday in June. This is considered to be the perfect color spectrum.

Near vision See **myopia**.

Ortho-K (OK) lenses These are hard contact lenses that are worn overnight for the purpose of reshaping the cornea, thus producing a temporary improvement in visual acuity. This practice, also known as orthokeratology, does not prevent myopia and it is associated with potentially dangerous side effects, such as corneal ulcers brought on by infection. These lenses are mostly sold within Chinese communities.

Ophthalmologist Medical doctor (M.D.) specializing in surgery and diseases of the eyes.

Optic center The precise center point of a lens (either minus or plus) which offers the optimum visual correction. Usually, the optic center point is placed directly in front of the eye when looking straight ahead. If the optic center is not positioned correctly the glasses will cause eyestrain.

If glasses are used for reading as well as for distance, especially those with higher diopter lenses, there will be a prism effect when reading. This means the eye will have to use additional convergence or divergence power to keep the image clear. This can potentially lead to convergence problems and fatigue. It is better to have different glasses prescribed for specific purposes – for instance, reading glasses should have a different prescription to glasses for computer work. This is because varying distances and angles of view must be taken into consideration.

Optometrist A specialist in measuring eyesight. They correct vision problems by prescribing glasses.

Phoria The tendency for either a horizontal or vertical misalignment of the eyes, which causes double vision, either near or far. It is tested using a Maddox prism.

Pseudomyopia Pseudomyopia refers to an occasional period of blurred distance vision, in most cases due to excessive near work such as reading or schoolwork.

Pursuit movements This refers to eye movements when reading: the eyes are supposed to follow the line that is being read. If pursuit movements are not smooth, then the child will regress and read the same line again. Or, if the convergence point moves in or out for each word (**fixation**), this will make reading extremely slow and tiring.

Retinoscope An instrument used to accurately determine focusing ability, which involves reflecting a light into the eye. Retinoscopy is the least disruptive way to test small children because it can be performed at a distance. It is also considered the most effective method available.

Saccadic eye movements When the eye moves from one word to another, the eyes are performing a saccadic movement. If the saccadic movement is not accurate, the child may lose their place in the text and read above or below the line they are supposed to be reading. Sometimes small two or three letter words fall away because the eyes simply miss them.

Scan The ability of the eye to look at letters, words and groups of words and gain information (visual attention). Children lacking this skill tend to guess words and have a hard time learning the alphabet.

Short sight See **myopia**.

Snellen chart This is the common eye-chart used either at 3 meters or 6 meters to check visual acuity at a distance.

Strabismus Where one eye turns in (esotropia) or out (exotropia). It requires special Vision Training or, in some cases, surgery.

Visagraph The Visagraph is a mask containing electronics that can detect very precise eye movements as the child reads. The result is output to a computer that shows the exact movements of the eye. This is by far the most effective way of testing eye movements. It is a five minute process that should be carried out before a child starts school, and ideally every year in primary school, so that any eye movement issues can be addressed without delay.

Vision Therapy Vision Therapy, also known as Vision Training, is used to improve vision skills such as eye movement control and eye co-ordination. It involves a series of exercises, usually under supervision by an orthoptist or optometrist.

Visual processing skills A set of skills that enable the brain to use information deduced from what the child can see. Problems in this area are linked to many reading and learning problems including visual dyslexia, dysgraphia and dyscalculia. There are a number of visual information processing sub-skills.

Bibliography

Allen, M. (n.d.). How to eliminate hyperopia. *International Society for the Enhancement of Eyesight*. Available at: http://www.i-see.org/allen_hyp.html.

American Optometric Association (2008). *Care of the Patient with Hyperopia. Optometric Clinical Practice Guideline*. St. Louis, MO: AOA.

Ashby, R., Ohlendorf, A. and Schaeffel, F. (2009). The effect of ambient illuminance on the development of deprivation myopia in chicks. *Investigative Ophthalmology & Visual Science* 50(11): 5348–5354.

Atkinson, J., Anker, S., Bobier, W., Braddick, O., Durden, K., Nardini, M. and Watson, P. (2000). Normal emmetropization in infants with spectacle correction for hyperopia. *Investigative Ophthalmology & Visual Science* 84: 181–188.

Atkinson, J., Braddick, O., Bobier, B., Anker, S., Ehrlich, D., King, J., Watson, P. and Moore, A. (1996). Two infant vision screening programs: predictions and prevention of strabismus and amblyopia from photo and video refractive screening. *Eye* 10: 189–198.

Augsburger, A. R. (1987). Hyperopia. In J. F. Amos (ed.), *Diagnosis and Management in Vision Care*. Boston, MA: Butterworths, pp. 101–119.

Bates, W. H. (1915). The cure of defective eyesight by treatment without glasses. *New York Medical Journal* 101(19): 925–933.

Bücklers, M. (1953). Changes in refraction during life. *British Journal of Ophthalmology* 37: 587–592.

Chryssanthou, G. (1974). Orthoptic management of intermittent exotropia. *American Orthoptic Journal* 24: 69–72.

Cotter, S. A. (2007). Management of childhood hyperopia: a pediatric optometrist's perspective. *Optometry and Vision Science* 84: 103–109.

Crane, A. and Crane, V. (2006). *Reading Problems Resolved: Helping Today's Children Read Proficiently for a Better Tomorrow*. Lions Crane Reading Program. Available at: http://www.ruidosonoonlions.org/foundations/reading%20problems%20resolved%20-%20pdf.pdf.

De Angelis, D. (2005). *How I Cured My Myopia: Prevent and Reverse Nearsightedness without Glasses, Contact Lenses and Surgery*. Bloomington, IN: iUniverse.

Donahue, S. P. (2004). How often are spectacles prescribed to "normal" preschool children? *Journal for American Association for Pediatric Ophthalmology and Strabismus* 8(3): 224–229.

Donders, F. C. (1864). *On the Anomalies of Accommodation and Refraction of the Eye*. Tr. W. D. Moore. London: New Sydenham Society.

Etting, G. (1978). Strabismus therapy in private practice: cure rates after three months of therapy. *Journal of the American Optometric Association* 49: 1367–1373.

Gwiazda, J. (2009). Treatment options for myopia. *Optometry and Vision Science* 86(6): 624–628.

Harb, E., Thorn, F. and Troilo, D. (2006). Characteristics of accommodative behaviour during sustained reading in emmotropes and myopes. *Vision Research* 46: 2581–2592.

Haro, C., Poulain, I. and Drobe, B. (2000). Investigation of working distance in myopic and non-myopic children. *Optometry and Vision Science* 77 (12, Suppl.): 189.

Hirsch, M. J. (1952). The changes in refraction between the ages of 5 and 14; theoretical and practical considerations. *American Journal of Optometry & Archives of American Academy of Optometry* 29(9): 445–459.

Hoffman, L. J. (1986). Incidence of vision difficulties in children with learning disabilities. *Journal of the American Optometric Association* 57: 44–55.

Hung, L. F., Crawford, M. L. and Smith, E. L. (1995). Spectacle lenses alter eye growth and the refractive status of young monkeys. *Nature Medicine* 1: 761–765.

Hutcheson, K. A., Ellish, N. J. and Lambert, S. R. (2003). Weaning children with accommodative esotropia out of spectacles: a pilot study. *British Journal of Ophthalmology* 87(1): 4–7.

Huxley, A. (1942). *The Art of Seeing: An Adventure in Reeducation.* New York: Harper and Row.

Ingram, R. M., Gill, L. E. and Lambert, T. W. (2000). Effect of spectacles on changes of spherical hypermetropia in infants who did, and did not, have strabismus. *British Journal of Ophthalmology* 84: 324–326.

Ingram, R. M., Arnold, P. E., Dally, S. et al. (1990). Results of randomised trial of treating abnormal hypermetropia from the age of 6 months. *British Journal of Ophthalmology* 74: 158–159.

Institut für Qualität und Wirtschaftlichkeit im Gesundheitswesen (2008). *Früherkennungsuntersuchung von Sehstörungen bei Kindern bis zur Vollendung des 6: Lebensjahres. Dokumentation und Würdigung der Stellungnahmen zum Vorbericht.* IQWIG: Köln.

Lie, I. (1989). Visual anomalies, visually related problems and reading difficulties. *Optometrie* 4: 15–20.

Mainstone, J. C., Carney, L. G., Anderson, C. R., Clem, P. M., Stephensen, A. L. and Wilson, M. D. (1998). Corneal shape in hyperopia. *Clinical and Experimental Optometry* 81(3): 131–137.

Menacker, S. J. and Batshaw, M. L. (1977). Vision: our window to the world. In M. L. Batshaw (ed.), *Children with Disabilities: A Medical Primer.* Baltimore, ML: Paul H. Brookes Publishing, 1997, pp. 220–221.

Meyer, E., Mizrahi, E. and Perlman, I. (1991). Amblyopia Success Index: a new method of quantitative assessment of treatment efficacy; applications in a study of 473 anisometropic amblyopic patients. *Binocular Vision & Strabismus Quarterly* 6: 75–82.

Napper, G. A., Brennan, N. A., Barrington, M., Squires, M. A., Vessey, G. A. and Vingrys, A. J. (1995). The duration of normal visual exposure necessary to prevent form deprivation myopia in chicks. *Vision Research* 35: 1337–1344.

Parssinen, O. and Lyyra, A. (1993). Myopia and myopia progression among school children: a three-year follow-up study. *Investigative Ophthalmology & Visual Science* 34(9): 2794–2802.

Rosenberg, R. (1991). Static retinoscopy. In J. B. Eskridge, J. F. Amos and J. D. Barlett (eds.), *Clinical Procedures in Optometry*. Philadelphia, PA: JB Lippincott, pp. 155–167.

Rosenfield, M. and Chin, N. N. (1995). Repeatability of subjective and objective refraction. *Optometry and Vision Science* 72: 577–579.

Rosner, J. and Gruber, J. (1985). Differences in the perceptual skills development of young myopes and hyperopes. *American Journal of Optometry and Physiological Optics* 62: 501–504.

Rosner, M. and Belkin, M. (1987). Intelligence, education and myopia in males. *Archives of Ophthalmology* 105: 1508–1511.

Schaeffel, F. (2009). Augenheilkunde–kurzsichtigkeitforschung – myopie. *Labor & More*. Available at: http://www.laborundmore.de/archive/226343/Augenheilkunde-Kurzsichtigkeitsforschung-Myopie.html/.

Schaeffel, F., Glasser, A. and Howland, H. C. (1988). Accommodation, refractive error and eye growth in chickens. *Vision Research* 28(5): 639–657.

Seet, B., Wong, T. Y., Tan, D. T., Saw, S. M., Balakrishnan, V., Lee, L. K. and Lim, A. S. (2001). Myopia in Singapore: taking a public health approach. *British Journal of Ophthalmology* 85(5): 521–526.

Smith III, E. L., Hung, L. F. and Harwerth, R. S. (1994). Effects of optically induced blur on the refractive status of young monkeys. *Vision Research* 34: 293–301.

Smith III, E. L., (1998). Spectacle lenses and emmetropization: the role of optical defocus in regular ocular development. *Optometry and Vision Science* 75(6): 388–398.

Smith III, E. L., and Hung, L. F. (1999). The role of optical defocus in regulating refractive development in infant monkeys. *Vision Research* 39: 1415–1435.

Stewart, C. E., Moseley, M. J., Stephens, D. A. and Fielder, A. R. (2004). Treatment dose-response in amblyopia therapy: the Monitored Occlusion Treatment of Amblyopia Study (MOTAS). *Investigative Ophthalmology & Visual Science* 45(9): 3048–3054.

Suchoff, I. B. and Petito, G. T. (1986). The efficacy of visual therapy: accommodative disorders and non-strabismic anomalies of binocular vision. *Journal of the American Optometric Association* 57(2): 119–125.

Tong, L., Huang, X. L., Koh, A. L., Zhang, X., Tan, D. T. and Chua, W. H. (2009). Atropine for the treatment of childhood myopia: effect on myopia progression after cessation of atropine. *Ophthalmology* 116(3): 572–579.

Villarreal, M. G., Ohlsson, J., Abrahamsson, M., Sjostrom, A. and Sjostrand, J. (2000). Myopisation: the refractive tendency in teenagers. Prevalence of myopia in young teenagers in Sweden. *Acta Ophthalmologica Scandinavica* 78(2): 177–181.

Wallman, J. and Winawer, J. (2004). Homeostasis of eye growth and the question of myopia. *Neuron* 43: 447–468.

Wick, B. (1987). Accommodative esotropia: efficacy of therapy. *Journal of the American Optometric Association* 58: 562–566.

Wick, B., Wingard, M., Cotter, S. and Scheiman, M. (1992). Anisometropic amblyopia: is the patient ever too old to treat? *Optometry and Vision Science* 69(11): 866–878.

Worth, C. (1903). *Squint: Its Causes, Pathology and Treatment.* Philadelphia, PA: Blackiston.

Young, F. A., Leary, G. A., Baldwin, W. R., West, D. C., Box, R. A., Harris, E. and Johnson, C. (1969). The transmission of refractive errors within Eskimo families. *American Journal of Optometry & Archives of American Academy of Optometry* 46(9): 676–685.

Zadnik, K., Mutti, D. O. and Adams, A. J. (1992). The repeatability of measurements of the ocular components. *Investigative Ophthalmology & Visual Science* 33: 2325–2333.

Zhu, X., Winawer, J. A. and Wallman, J. (2003). Potency of myopic defocus in spectacle lens compensation. *Investigative Ophthalmology & Visual Science* 44: 2818–2827.

Zylbermann, R., Landau, D. and Berson, D. (1993). The influence of study habits on myopia in Jewish teenagers. *Journal of Pediatric Ophthalmology & Strabismus* 30(5): 319–322.

List of charts and exercises

Charts

Charts can be downloaded from: http://www.vision-training. com/en/Download/Download.html.

Exercises

About the Author

Leo Angart was born in Denmark and has lived in Asia for more than 30 years. For most of that time he lived in Hong Kong. Currently he is based in Munich. Leo wore glasses for more than 26 years before he discovered how to regain his normal eyesight in 1991. The remarkable thing about his recovery is that it was accomplished through methods outside the traditional vision improvement methods.

Leo has combined his knowledge of neurolinguistic programming with many years of experience helping people to regain their eyesight. He has distilled his methodology into simple exercises specific to particular problems. Most importantly, the exercises give quick results.

Since 1996 Leo has conducted his weekend Vision Training workshops more than 25 times every year in major cities around the world. His workshops fill up quickly because they provide the how of Vision Training. Leo will give you the motivation and the specific steps. You, in turn, are responsible for doing the exercises. The encouraging part is that you will see an improvement almost immediately.

There is more information at www.vision-training.com.

If you would like to attend one of Leo's workshops, please check the schedule on the website to find a workshop near you.